Consensus Development in Cancer Therapy 1

Consensus Development in Cancer Therapy 1

Therapeutic Management of Metastatic Breast Cancer

Editors
M. Kaufmann, I. C. Henderson, E. Enghofer

Walter de Gruyter
Berlin · New York 1989

Editors

PD Dr. M. Kaufmann
Universitäts-Frauenklinik
Vößstr. 9
D-6900 Heidelberg
FRG

Prof. Dr. I. C. Henderson
Dana-Farber Cancer Institute
Division of Medical Oncology
44 Binney Street
Boston, MA 02115
USA

Dr. E. Enghofer
Wessobrunner Str. 5
D-8032 Gräfelfing
FRG

Deutsche Bibliothek Cataloging-in-Publication Data

Therapeutic management of metastatic breast cancer / ed. M. Kaufmann ... [First named authors: K. W. Brunner ...]. – Berlin ; New York : de Gruyter, 1989
(Consensus development in cancer therapy ; 1)
ISBN 3-11-012182-4
NE: Kaufmann, Manfred [Hrsg.]: GT

Library of Congress Cataloging-in-Publication Data

Therapeutic management of metastatic breast cancer / editors, M. Kaufmann, I. C. Henderson, E. Enghofer.
p. cm. – (Consensus development in cancer therapy ; 1)
Proceedings of a conference.
ISBN 0-89925-607-4
1. Breast – Cancer – Treatment – Congresses. 2. Metastasis – Congresses. I. Kaufmann, M. (Manfred), 1946- . II. Henderson, I. Craig. III. Enghofer, E. (Erich), 1949- . IV. Series.
[DNLM: 1. Breast Neoplasms – therapy – congresses. 2. Neoplasm Metastasis – congresses. WP 870 T3975]
RC280.B8T46 1989
616.99′44906 – dc20
DNLM/DLC

 Typesetting: Arthur Collignon GmbH, Berlin. – Printing: Gerike GmbH, Berlin. – Binding: Lüderitz & Bauer GmbH, Berlin. – Cover design: Rudolf Hübler, Berlin. – Printed in Germany.

First-named authors

Prof. Dr. K. W. Brunner
Inselhospital Bern
Institut für Med. Onkologie
der Universität
CH-3010 Bern
Switzerland

Dr. R. C. Coombes
Clinical Oncology Unit
St. George's Hospital
Medical School
Grammer Terrace
London SW17 ORE
UK

Prof. Dr. I. C. Henderson
Dana-Farber Cancer Institute
Division of Medical Oncology
44 Binney Street
Boston, MA 02115
USA

PD Dr. M. Kaufmann
Universitäts-Frauenklinik
Vößstr. 9
D-6900 Heidelberg
FRG

Prof. Dr. A. Neiß
Institut für Biostatistik
Universität Innsbruck
Müllerstr. 59/II
A-6010 Innsbruck
Austria

PD Dr. K. Possinger
Med. Klinik III,
Klinikum Großhadern
Ludwig-Maximilians-Universität
Marschioninistr. 15
D-8000 München 70
FRG

Dr. C. Rose
Department of Oncology R
Odense University Hospital
DK-5000 Odense C
Denmark

Prof. J. E. Smith, M. D.
Royal Marsden Hospital
Fulham Road
London SW3 6JJ
UK

Contents

Introduction

As a consequence of the Consensus Conference in Washington (Sept. 1985) and a Symposium in St. Gallen, Switzerland, (March 1988) well defined standard guidelines for adjuvant treatment of breast cancer were set.

For palliative treatment of metastatic breast cancer, very different approaches are taken and a concise evaluation from a scientific point of view was missing.

M. Kaufmann, Heidelberg, and I. C. Henderson, Boston, chaired a Consensus Development Conference on July 8 – 9, 1988 in Munich which dealt with "Therapeutic Management of Metastatic Breast Cancer".*

The experts who took part in this International Conference were from different medical departments and came from West Germany, Austria, Switzerland, Denmark, the U.K. and America. The situation in Germany was given special consideration.

The Consensus Statement is a comprehensive overview on the state-of-the-art knowledge of the palliative treatment of breast cancer. It should provide a guideline for the therapeutic management both within and outside of the clinic; it cannot, however, provide answers to questions which have yet to be clarified in the framework of further clinical trials.

The editors

---

* Supported by Lederle Laboratories, Wolfratshausen, Germany.

Endocrine therapy of advanced breast cancer

C. Rose

Abstract

Recent research has resulted in several new options for endocrine treatment of advanced breast cancer. Since one of the most intriguing characteristics of endocrine therapy is that new remissions can be acheived when using subsequent endocrine modalities, it is of importance to evaluate their optimal sequence. Tamoxifen has become the most commonly used endocrine therapy of advanced breast cancer due to its few side effects and an overall response rate of 35%, which has been obtained in randomized trials of tamoxifen compared with either ablative, additive or inhibitive treatment approaches. Crossover data from these trials indicate that the highest overall response rate is obtained when tamoxifen is used as first line endocrine therapy. Furthermore, it seems that oophorectomy in premenopausal and aminoglutethimide or progestins in postmenopausal patients are equally effective as second line endocrine therapy.

Despite an obvious clinical rationale for combined endocrine therapy, most trials exploring this concept have failed to show any benefit. Although data from trials combining tamoxifen with prednisolone or androgens seem exciting, the use of combined endocrine therapy still has to be considered experimental.

Introduction

Treatment of advanced breast cancer is palliative. Optimal efficacy of cytotoxic therapy has been reached by achieving response rates of 60% and median times to progression of 8 – 12 months. This has resulted in a renewed interest in the various endocrine therapies used either alone, in combination with each other or in addition to multiple cytotoxic therapy. Recently, a number of trials have demonstrated that endocrine therapy with tamoxifen followed by cytotoxic therapy upon progression is as effective in terms of overall response rate and survival as cytotoxic treatment and tamoxifen given simultaneously or sequentially to postmenopausal patients with advanced breast cancer [5, 37, 1, 46, 50].

One of the characteristics of the various forms of endocrine therapy is that a response can be predicted by the presence of estrogen and/or progesterone receptors in patients' tumor tissue. All the different endocrine modalities have a lower acute toxicity and a lower long term morbidity than the cytotoxic approaches. Moreover, one of the most intriguing characteristics of endocrine therapy is that subsequent remissions can be obtained with successive endocrine therapies. It is therefore of clinical importance to evaluate whether there is an optimal sequence in which these therapies can be administered. A rational approach to such an evaluation would be the execution of carefully designed phase III studies in receptor positive patients with a crossover of all patients upon progression. No such trials have ever been performed. We are therefore forced to analyse data from anecdotal reports, phase II trials and comparative trials with crossover data from a minority of the patients. Several comprehensive reviews have been published in which available data have been pooled [12, 45, 36, 40, 26] (table 1). There are, however, objections to this approach. Different criteria for response have been used to access the outcome of therapy and different selection criteria for patients have evolved with time. Furthermore, prognostic variables are not equally represented in the different trials and since most of the data in these reviews stem from phase II trials in which determination of response rate is the only aim, valid knowledge about time to progression is not available. Moreover, data on cross sensitivity and non-cross resistance are not necessarily reliable due to a possible withdrawal response. These problems can partly be overcome by a restriction of the analysis to randomized trials in which a minority of the patients have been crossed over to treatment with the comparative therapy.

The efficacy and low toxicity of tamoxifen have been established in comparative trials with other ablative, additive, or inhibitive treatment approaches [37].

Table 1 Response data from comprehensive reviews

Therapy	N	Response rate (%)	Reference
Ablative			
Ovx	1674	33	Henderson [12]
Adx	3739	32	Henderson [12]
Hypx	1174	36	Henderson [12]
Inhibitive			
Ag + H	1153	31	Stuart-Harris [45]
Additive			
Estrogens	1683	26	Henderson [12]
Progestins	1746	29	Rose [36]
Androgens	2250	21	Henderson [12]
Glucocorticoids	756	25	Santen [40]
Competitive			
Tamoxifen	1269	32	Mouridsen [40]

Although none of these trials have included a large enough number of patients to allow detection of even great differences in response rate (10–20%), these trials have been of prime importance in placing tamoxifen as the treatment of choice for first line endocrine therapy. Furthermore, a number of trials have explored the possibility of an increased efficacy by combining tamoxifen with other endocrine approaches.

In the following we will therefore first analyse data from trials between tamoxifen and other endocrine therapies. Secondly, we will review trials of combined endocrine therapy where tamoxifen is used as one of the endocrine modalities.

Material

All randomized trials reviewed here meet the following selection criteria:

1. at least 20 patients in each treatment group,
2. similar response criteria,
3. information concerning relevant data such as response rate, toxicity, time to progression, and survival.

In the analysis of the trials we have focused upon treatment efficacy and side effects.

Efficacy of endocrine therapy

The efficacy of the various endocrine therapies can be assessed by considering time to progression, response rate, and crossover data (cross sensitivity and non-cross resistance). Furthermore, treatment efficacy can be evaluated in relation to prognostic factors such as, for example, estrogen receptor (ER) status. Since only a few studies give data regarding time to progression, only response rates will be compared within the various trials.

Tamoxifen has been compared with other endocrine modalities in 26 randomized trials which are summarized in table 2. Premenopausal patients have been randomized to either tamoxifen or oophorectomy in 2 trials [16, 4]. Both yielded similar response rates and revealed no major differences in other treatment endpoints. Adrenalectomy vs. tamoxifen has been compared in a single trial [29]. A non-significant difference in response rate in favour of adrenalectomy was obtained. A rate of response in the order of 30–35% has been found, regardless of whether treatment has been tamoxifen, aminoglutethimide and hydrocortison [42, 20], estrogens [43, 13, 33, 10, 2, 22], medroxyprogesterone acetate (MPA) [34, 3, 30, 8, 49, 41, 21, 9] or megestrole acetate (MA) [14, 24, 6, 27]. In the 3 trials analysing the relative efficacy of androgens vs. tamoxifen [52, 28, 17] there is a trend towards a lower response rate for patients treated with androgens as first line endocrine therapy.

Table 2 Response to tamoxifen compared to other endocrine modalities in advanced breast cancer. Summary of 26 randomized trials.

No. of trials	Tamoxifen N	(%)	Comparative therapy N	(%)	
2	81	(25)	79	(27)	Ovx
1	26	(35)	25	(52)	Adx
6	248	(27)	249	(28)	Estrogens
3	123	(26)	136	(18)	Androgens
12	696	(34)	762	(35)	Progestins
2	99	(33)	93	(32)	AG + H

Crossover data

It is important to evaluate the cross sensitivity and non-cross resistance (table 3) between two endocrine treatment modalities given sequentially, since such infor-

Table 3 Terminology of crossover data

<table>
<tr><td colspan="2" rowspan="2"></td><td colspan="2">1. line therapy</td></tr>
<tr><td>R</td><td>NR</td></tr>
<tr><td rowspan="2">2. line therapy</td><td>R</td><td>Cross Sensitivity</td><td>Non-cross Resistance</td></tr>
<tr><td>NR</td><td>Non-cross Sensitivity</td><td>Cross Resistance</td></tr>
</table>

R: Responders NR: Non-responders

mation can elucidate the proper sequence of the various therapies. Table 4 shows the available data on cross sensitivity. Although the number of patients in each trial is small, it is obvious that the response rate to second line treatment with tamoxifen in patients who have responded to a previous endocrine treatment is lower than the response rate to any other second line endocrine therapy in patients who have first responded to tamoxifen. For patients who have not responded to first line endocrine therapy, the rate of response to second line therapy is essentially independent of treatment modality and is approximately 10% (table 5). There is, however, a tendency towards a higher rate of response when tamoxifen is given as the first therapy.

Table 4 Cross sensitivity between tamoxifen and other endocrine therapies

No. of trials	Response to TAM in responders to comparative ET		Response to comparative ET in responders to TAM		
	N	(%)	N	(%)	
1	7	(14)	5	(40)	Ovx
1	6	(17)	2	(50)	Adx
4	11	(36)	22	(36)	Estrogens
5	15	(13)	27	(33)	Progestins
3	20	(25)	26	(39)	Ag + H

Table 5 Non-cross resistance between tamoxifen and other endocrine therapies

No. of trials	Response to TAM in non-responders to comparative ET		Response to comparative ET in non-responders to TAM		
	N	(%)	N	(%)	
1	11	(9)	10	(30)	Ovx
1	9	(22)	7	(57)	Adx
4	52	(21)	41	(17)	Estrogens
1	20	(15)	10	(10)	Androgens
5	53	(6)	104	(10)	Progestins
3	42	(7)	61	(12)	AG + H

Response and ER-status

Only a few of the randomized phase III studies we are considering here have correlated the response to endocrine therapy with the presence of ER. In all these studies, only a small subset of the total group of patients had ER-analysis performed, and the different investigators have used different techniques and cut-off limits. Furthermore, none of these studies distinguish between receptor analysis performed on tumor tissue from the primary tumor vs. that from a metastasis. The response rate in ER-positive patients range from 0–57% in the various studies. In the corresponding ER-negative group the response rate is only about 10%. However, it is of importance for this analysis that response rate in relation to ER-status seems to be independent of the form of endocrine therapy used.

Side-effects or problems with endocrine therapy

The only reliable comparison between the different endocrine therapies with regard to side-effects would have to be based upon knowledge of the number of patients, who had to discontinue treatment, or who had to have the dose reduced. Only a few of the trials analysed herein give such information. Furthermore, the toxicity profiles are so different from the various therapies that a direct comparison is almost meaningless. A more or less subjective assessment must therefore be given. Since the surgical procedures are irreversible, they have to be restricted to those patients with a relatively high probability of response. Side-effects from treatment with estrogens or androgens in the form of congestive heart failure and/or virilization are considered by many to be more serious than the lethargy or fluid retention recorded in patients treated with aminoglutethimide or a progestin.

Relative cost of endocrine therapies

Based upon analysis of the relative efficacy of the various endocrine treatment modalities and their toxicity, it seems justified that tamoxifen currently is considered the drug of choice for first line endocrine therapy. However, all societies have to be concerned about the cost-effectiveness of medical treatments of nearly identical efficacy and toxicity. In order to be able to compare ablative procedures with pharmacological therapies, we have therefore estimated the cost of a response to various endocrine therapies in both the UK and in Denmark. Based upon a response rate of 35% for the various therapies and a median time to progression of 8 months it seems that surgical procedures are expensive in comparison with any pharmacological treatment. When only the latter therapies are compared it appears that the cost of a response obtained with MPA and the LHRH-agonists Buserelin or Zoladex is about 3–5 times that obtained either by aminoglutethimide and hydrocortisone, MA, halotestin (HAL), or tamoxifen. Without exception, even high doses of diethylstilbestrol (DES) is the most inexpensive treatment of all pharmacological therapies of breast cancer. As a further example, the price for tamoxifen is about 7 times that of DES in the United States. Finally, it can be shown that the cost of a response obtained by actinic castration is in the same order as pharmacological treatment with HAL or tamoxifen.

Evaluation of the possible candidates for endocrine therapy in pre- and postmenopausal advanced breast cancer

On the basis of the relative efficacy, side effects and price, the various options for endocrine therapy of pre- and postmenopausal advanced breast cancer will be considered separately.

Premenopausal advanced breast cancer

Castration, either by surgery or by irradiation, is the oldest form of endocrine therapy, and until recently it was considered to be the treatment of choice in all premenopausal patients with metastatic disease. The overall response rate in 1674 premenopausal patients was 33% [12]. Surgical or actinic castration have never been compared in a randomized trial. However, actinic castration has produced similar rates of response as those obtained by oophorectomy [7, 19]. It is therefore reasonable to believe that ovarian ablation by radiotherapy can substitute the surgical procedures due to comparable efficacy and a lower cost. Rather high doses of estrogens have been tried in premenopausal patients and seem to be without effect [18]. Androgens can be used to induce menostasia, but this requires high doses, which in most cases lead to unacceptable virilization. Table 6 shows in greater details the only 2 randomized comparisons between tamoxifen and oophorectomy. Although the numbers are small, similar rates of response are obtained and none of the two studies demonstrate any difference in survival.

Table 6 Randomized trials comparing tamoxifen with oophorectomy in advanced breast cancer

References	Treatment (daily dose)	Response rate (CR + PR)/N	(%)	Response duration++ (days)	Time to treatment failure++ (days)	Survival++ (days)
Ingle [16]	TAM (20 mg)	7/26	(27%)	453	160	749
	Oophorectomy	10/27	(37%)	476	144	722
Buchanan [4]	TAM (40 mg)	13/55	(24%)	600	–	450
	Oophorectomy	11/52	(21%)	210	–	750

++ – median

Table 7 Randomized trials comparing tamoxifen and estrogens in advanced breast cancer

References	Treatment	(daily dose)	Response rate (CR + PR)/N	(%)	Response duration++ (days)	Time to treatment failure++ (days)	Survival++ (days)
Stewart [43]	TAM	(10 mg × 3)	9/29	(31%)	266	–	–
	DES	(5 mg × 3)	6/27	(22%)	228	–	–
Ingle [13]	TAM	(10 mg × 2)	23/69	(33%)	238	171	735
	DES	(5 mg × 3)	30/74	(41%)	393	142	1140
Ribeiro [33]	TAM	(20 mg)	13/47	(28%)	720	–	–
	DES	(3 mg)	14/45	(31%)	720	–	–
Gockerman [10]	TAM	(10 mg × 2)	3/54	(6%)	–	150	1020
	DES	(5 mg × 3)	5/50	(10%)	–	180	1050
Beex [2]	TAM	(20 mg × 2)	10/30	(33%)	330	–	750
	EE_2	(3 mg)	9/29	(31%)	360	–	930
Matelski [22]	TAM	(20 mg)	10/19	(53%)	–	–	–
	EE_2	(3 mg)	6/24	(25%)	–	–	–

++ – median

Postmenopausal advanced breast cancer

Because of the favourable cost-effective relationship for treatment with estrogens, the randomized comparisons between tamoxifen and DES or ethinylestradiol are summarized in table 7. It appears that the various treatment endpoints are comparable between the two treatment options and without significant differences. It is well known that estrogen therapies display a variety of toxicities. Although some of the side-effects of estrogen treatment are claimed to be less severe with continued treatment, it is clearly demonstrated in all 6 randomized trials that the toxicity of tamoxifen is milder and generally without importance. In addition, treatment with estrogens had to be discontinued due to side-effects in about 50% of patients in two of the trials [43, 22]. Even in the study by Ribeiro [33] using only 3 mg of DES daily, 15% of the patients had to stop treatment. Nevertheless even such a substantial proportion of patients stopping treatment because of side-effects did not seem to influence the therapeutic outcome of treatment with estrogens.

Combined endocrine therapy

The clinical experience of partial cross sensitivity and a lack of complete cross resistance between the different endocrine treatment modalities indicate that these therapies may not share the same ultimate modes of action [37]. Thus there is a rationale for the simultaneous application of the different endocrine therapies. In Denmark, we have performed 3 randomized clinical trials, comparing treatment with tamoxifen alone and tamoxifen in combination with either additive or inhibitive endocrine treatment in postmenopausal patients with advanced breast cancer [26, 38].

The results from these 3 trials in postmenopausal patients with progressive breast cancer demonstrated that first line endocrine therapy with tamoxifen was just as effective as treatment with tamoxifen in combination with either MPA, DES, aminoglutethimide and hydrocortisone or HAL. Toxicity was more pronounced and severe in the combined treatment groups in all three trials.

Other investigators have explored the effect of combined endocrine therapy in randomized trials and the results of combining tamoxifen with an androgen or aminoglutethimide and hydrocortisone are shown in table 8 and 9, respectively. In four out of five trials analysing the addition of androgen to tamoxifen, a trend for an increased response rate is demonstrated. Preliminary data from the largest of these trials [51] even suggest a survival advantage for the combined approach.

The addition of aminoglutethimide and hydrocortisone to tamoxifen has been analysed in four trials (table 8). By combining both tamoxifen, aminoglutethim-

Table 8 Randomized trials of tamoxifen in combination with androgens in advanced breast cancer

References	Treatment (daily dose)		Response rate (CR + PR)/N	(%)	Response duration++ (days)	Time to treatment failure++ (days)	Survival++ (days)
Tormey [47]	TAM	(2 – 100 mg/m^2 × 2)	8/52	(15%)	230	64	330
	TAM	(2 – 100 mg/m^2 × 2)	21/56	(37%)	212	180	380
	FLU	(7 mg/m^2 × 2)					
Twito [48]	TAM	(10 mg × 2)	50/119	(42%)	–	199	860
	TAM	(10 mg × 2)	62/120	(52%)	–	364	917
	FLU	(10 mg × 2)					
Rose [35]	TAM	(10 mg × 3)	32/94	(34%)	720	300	720
	TAM	(10 mg × 3)	36/87	(44%)	720	330	720
	FLU	(5 mg × 4)					
Wallgren [51]	TAM	(20 mg × 2)	36/145	(25%)	615	–	696
	TAM	(20 mg × 2)	51/139	(37%)	>720	–	964
	FLU	(10 mg × 2)					
Heinonen [11]	TAM	(10 mg × 3)	24/49	(49%)	–	390	870
	TAM	(10 mg × 3)	22/49	(45%)	–	360	750
	NAND	(100 mg i. m./w./2. w.)					

++ – median

Table 9 Randomized trials of tamoxifen in combination with inhibitive endocrine therapy or glucocorticoids in advanced breast cancer

References	Therapy (daily dose)		Response rate (CR + PR)/N	(%)	Response duration++ (days)	Time to treatment failure++ (days)	Survival++ (days)
Powles [32]	TAM	(10 mg × 2)	34/111	(31%)	675	–	1440 CR + PR
	TAM	(10 mg × 2)					
	AG + H	(250 mg × 3 + 20 mg × 2)	48/111	(43%)	540	–	690 CR + PR
	Danazol	(100 mg × 3)					
Milsted [23]	TAM	(10 mg × 2)	5/26	(19%)	–	–	–
	TAM	(10 mg × 2)					
	AG + H	(250 mg × 4 + 10 mg × 2)	6/26	(23%)	–	–	–
Ingle [15]	TAM	(10 mg × 2)	21/49	(43%)	452	216	657
	TAM	(10 mg × 2)					
	AG + H	(250 mg × 4 + 100 mg ⟶ 40)	25/51	(49%)	447	227	827
Rose [35]	TAM	(10 mg × 3)	32/94	(34%)	720	300	720
	TAM	(10 mg × 3)					
	AG + H	(250 mg × 4 + 20 mg × 3)	24/83	(29%)	720	240	720
Stewart [44]	TAM	(10 mg × 2)	9/72	(13%)	390	–	360
	TAM	(10 mg × 2)	26/73	(36%)	390	–	630
	Pred.	(5 mg × 2)					
Rubens [39]	TAM	(10 mg × 2)	24/77	(31%)+	360	–	NS
	TAM	(10 mg × 2)	39/85	(46%)+	720	–	NS
	Pred.	(5 mg × 2)					

++ – median + – ref.: R. D. Rubens: Personal communication NS – not significant ide, hydrocortisone and danazole, Powles et al. [32] obtained a 12% increase in response rate. However, this increase was not translated into a prolongation of either response duration or survival. The addition of prednisolone to tamoxifen has been demonstrated to increase the response rate in two consecutive trials performed by the same group [44, 39]. Based upon the results in these two trials it can be predicted that the response rate to tamoxifen in combination with prednisolone will be 10 – 40% higher than to tamoxifen alone. In the latter trial, it appears from a preliminary analysis that the higher rate of response was translated into a prolongation of time to progression and survival.

Conclusion

Considering efficacy, side-effects, and cost of the various options for single agent endocrine therapy, and assuming that every patient with metastatic disease should have at least one trial of endocrine therapy, it seems justified that tamoxifen is the treatment of choice for first line endocrine therapy in both pre- and postmenopausal breast cancer patients. Current knowledge about cross sensitivity and price suggests that actinic castration among premenopausal women and aminoglutethimide and hydrocortisone or MA for postmenopausal women is a reasonable choice for second line endocrine therapy in previous responders to tamoxifen. If third line endocrine therapy is to be considered, aminoglutethimide and hydrocortisone, MA or DES might be of use.

Despite an obvious clinical rationale for combined endocrine therapy most trials exploring this concept have failed to show any benefit. Although data from trials combining tamoxifen with prednisolone or an androgen seem exciting, the use of combined endocrine therapy cannot at present be recommended outside the context of randomized clinical trials.

References

[1] Australian and New Zealand Breast Cancer Trials Group. A randomized trial in postmenopausal patients with advanced breast cancer comparing endocrine and cytotoxic therapy given sequentially or in combination. J. Clin. Oncol. *4* (1986) 186.

[2] Beex, L., G. Pieters, A. Smals et al.: Tamoxifen Versus Ethinyl Estradiol in the Treatment of Postmenopausal Women With Advanced Breast Cancer. Cancer Treat. Rep. *65* (1981) 179.

[3] Beretta, G., D. Tabiadon, L. Tedeschi et al.: Hormonotherapy of Advanced Breast Carcinoma: Comparative Evaluation of Tamoxifen Citrate Versus Medroxyprogesterone Acetate. In: S. Iacobelli et al. (eds.): The Role of Tamoxifen in Breast Cancer, p. 113. Raven Press, New York 1982.

[4] Buchanan, R. B., R. W. Blamey, K. R. Durrant et al.: A Randomized Comparison of Tamoxifen With Surgical Oophorectomy in Premenopausal Patients With Advanced Breast Cancer. J. Clin. Oncol. *4* (1986) 1326.

[5] Cavalli, F., M. Beer, G. Martz et al.: Concurrent or sequential use of cytotoxic chemotherapy and hormone treatment in advanced breast cancer: Report of the Swiss Group for Clinical Cancer Research. Br. Med. J. *286* (1983) 5.

[6] Ettinger, D. S., J. Allegra, J. R. Bertino et al.: Megestrol Acetate v. Tamoxifen in Advanced Breast Cancer: Correlation of Hormone Receptors and Response. Sem. Oncol. *13* (suppl. 4) (1986) 9.

[7] Fitzpatrick, P. J., P. G. Garret: Metastatic breast cancer: ovarian ablation with lower half-body irradiation. Int. J. Radiat. Oncol. Biol. Phys. *7* (1981) 1523.

[8] Fosser, V.: MPA Breast-Cancer Italian Clinical Trial Group: A multicentre randomized clinical trial with medroxyprogesterone acetata (MPA) at two different dosage schedules versus Tamoxifen (TMX) in advanced breast cancer. Proc. 3rd Germ.-Ital. Oncol. Symp. (1984) 79.

[9] Garcia-Giralt, E., P. Hurteloup, P. Chollet et al.: Breast cancer first line hormonotherapy: A multicenter randomized trial comparing TAM with MAP & their sequential administration. Proceedings of ASCO 6 (1987) Abstr. 236, 61.

[10] Gockerman, J. P., E. N. Spremulli, M. Raney et al.: Randomized Comparison of Tamoxifen Versus Diethylstilbestrol in Estrogen Receptor-Positive or -Unknown Metastatic Breast Cancer: A Southeastern Cancer Study Group Trial. Cancer Treat. Rep. *70* (1986) 1199.

[11] Heinonen, E., A. Alanko, P. Gröhn et al.: Nandrolone decanoate added to tamoxifen in the treatment of advanced breast cancer. Breast Cancer Res. Treat. *5* (1985) 75.

[12] Henderson, I. C., G. P. Canellos: Cancer of the breast. The past decade. New Engl. J. Med. *302* (1980) 17 & 78.

[13] Ingle, J. N., D. L. Ahmann, S. J. Green et al.: Randomized Clinical Trial of Diethylstilbestrol Versus Tamoxifen in Postmenopausal Women with Advanced Breast Cancer. New Engl. J. Med. *304* (1981) 16.

[14] Ingle, J. N., D. L. Ahmann, S. J. Green et al.: Randomized clinical trial of megestrol acetate versus tamoxifen in paramenopausal or castrated women with advanced breast cancer. Am. J. Clin. Oncol. *5* (1982) 155.

[15] Ingle, J. N., S. J. Green, D. L. Ahmann et al.: Randomized Trial of Tamoxifen Alone or Combined With Aminoglutethimide and Hydrocortisone in Women With Metastatic Breast Cancer. J. Clin. Oncol. *4* (1986) 958.

[16] Ingle, J. N., J. E. Krook, S. J. Green et al.: Randomized Trial of Bilateral Oophorectomy Versus Tamoxifen in Premenopausal Women With Metastatic Breast Cancer. J. Clin. Oncol. *4* (1986) 178.

[17] Johansson, R., E. Nordman: Tamoxifen and Nandrolonedecanoate in Treatment of Metastatic Breast Cancer; a Randomized Study. Proceedings of the third EORTC Breast Cancer Conference. Amsterdam (1983) Abstr. IX, 18.

[18] Kennedy, B. J.: Massive estrogen administration in premenopausal women with metastatic breast cancer. Cancer *15* (1962) 641.

[19] Lee, Y.-T. N.: Therapeutic Castration for Advanced Breast Cancer. Am. J. Surg. *122* (1971) 42.

[20] Lipton, A., H. A. Harvey, R. J. Santen et al.: Randomized Trial of Aminoglutethimide versus Tamoxifen in Metastatic Breast Cancer. Cancer Res. *42* (suppl.) (1982) 3434 s.

[21] Lorenz, I., Z. Mechl: Medroxyprogesterone acetate versus tamoxifen in the therapy of advanced breast cancer. Neoplasma *32* (1985) 119.

[22] Matelski, H., M. Huberman, T. Zipoli et al.: Randomized trial of estrogen vs. tamoxifen therapy for advanced breast cancer. Am. J. Clin. Oncol. *8* (1985) 128.

[23] Milsted, R., T. Habeshaw, S. Kaye et al.: A randomized trial of tamoxifen versus tamoxifen with aminoglutethimide in postmenopausal women with advanced breast cancer. Cancer Chemother. Pharmacol. *14* (1985) 272.

[24] Morgan, L. R.: Megestrol Acetate v. Tamoxifen in Advanced Breast Cancer in Postmenopausal Patients. Sem. Oncol. *12* (suppl. 1) (1985) 43.

[25] Mouridsen, H. T., T. Palshof, J. Patterson et al.: Tamoxifen in advanced breast cancer. Cancer Treat. Rev. *5* (1978) 131.

[26] Mouridsen, H. T., T. Palshof, C. Rose: Therapeutic effect of tamoxifen alone versus tamoxifen in combination with gestagen and estrogen in advanced breast cancer. Recent Results Cancer Res. *71* (1980) 169.

[27] Muss, H., E. Paschold, W. Black et al.: Megestrol acetate (M) v. Tamoxifen (T) in advanced breast cancer (ABC): a five years report. ASCO *6* (1987) Abstr. 214, 55.

[28] Nagai, R., S. Kumaoka: Clinical Evaluation of Tamoxifen in Advanced Breast Cancer (Primary & Recurrent) – Double Blind Study –. Clin. Eval. *8* (1980) 321.

[29] Nemoto, T., J. Patel, D. Rosner et al.: Tamoxifen (Nolvadex) Versus Adrenalectomy in Metastatic Breast Cancer. Cancer *53* (1984) 1333.

[30] Pannuti, F., A. Martoni, F. Fruet et al.: Oral High Dose Medroxyprogesterone Acetate Versus Tamoxifen in Postmenopausal Patients with Advanced Breast Cancer. In: S. Iacobelli et al. (eds.): The Role of Tamoxifen in Breast Cancer, p. 85. Raven Press, New York 1982.

[31] Pouillart, P., M. Jouve, T. Palangie et al.: Metastatic breast cancer. Controlled trial studying the optimal timing of honomotherapy combined with chemotherapy (Preliminary report). ASCO *3* (1984) Abstr. C-505, 129.

[32] Powles, T. J., S. Ashley, H. T. Ford et al.: Teatment of disseminated breast cancer with tamoxifen, aminoglutethimide, hydrocortisone, and danazole, used in combination or sequentially. Lancet (1984) 1369.

[33] Ribeiro, G. G.: A Clinical Trial to Compare the Use of Tamoxifen v. Stilboestrol in the Treatment of Postmenopausal Women with Advanced Breast Cancer. Rev. on Endocrine-Related Cancer *9* (suppl.) (1981) 409.

[34] Robustelli, Cuna G. della: Tamoxifen Versus Medroxyprogesterone Acetate Loading Doses as a Third-Line Therapy for Pretreated Progressive Postmenopausal Breast Carcinoma. Cur. Chemotherapy & Immun. ther. *11* (1982) 1479.

[35] Rose, C., C. Kamby, H. T. Mouridsen, L. Bastholt et al.: Combined endocrine treatment of post menopausal patients with advanced breast cancer. ASCO *5* (1986) Abstr. 247, 64.

[36] Rose, C., J. Løber, H. T. Mouridsen: Treatment of advanced breast cancer with progestins. A review. (In preparation).

[37] Rose, C., H. T. Mouridsen: Treatment of Advanced Breast Cancer with Tamoxifen. Recent Results in Cancer Res. *91* (1984) 230.

[38] Rose, C., H. T. Mouridsen: Combined Endocrine Treatment of Postmenospausal Patients with Advanced Breast Cancer. The Danish Experience. Tumor Diagn. & Ther. *8* (1987) 279.

[39] Rubens, R. D., R. K. Knight: The contribution of prednisolone (P) to primary endocrine therapy (PET) in advanced breast cancer. ASCO *1* (1985) Abstr. C 202, 53.

[40] Santen, R. J., E. Samojlik: Medical Adrenalectomy for Treatment of Metastatic Breast Carcinoma, p. 79. In: W. L. McGuire (ed.): Breast Cancer: Advances in Research and Treatment. Plenum Medical Book Company, New York 1979.

[41] Silva, A.: Medroxyprogesterone Acetate versus Tamoxifen in Advanced Breast Cancer. Proc. 3rd ECCO. Stockholm (1985) poster 13338.

[42] Smith, I. E., A. L. Harris, M. Morgan et al.: Tamoxifen versus aminoglutethimide in advanced breast carcinoma: a randomised cross-over trial. Br. Med. J. *283* (1981) 1432.

[43] Stewart, H. J., A. P. M. Forrest, J. M. Gunn et al.: The Tamoxifen Trial – A Double-Blind Comparison with Stilboestrol in Postmenopausal Women with Advanced Breast Cancer. Eur. J. Cancer *1* (suppl.) (1980) 83.

[44] Stewart, J. F., R. D. Rubens, R. J. B. King et al.: Contribution of prednisolone to the primary endocrine treatment of advanced breast cancer. Eur. J. Cancer Clin. Oncol. *18* (1982) 1307.

[45] Stuart-Harris, R. C., I. E. Smith: Aminoglutethimide in the treatment of advanced breast cancer. Cancer Treat. Rev. *11* (1984) 189.

[46] Taylor, S. G., R. S. Gelman, G. Falkson et al.: Combination chemotherapy compared to tamoxifen as initial therapy for stage IV breast cancer in elderly women. Ann. Intern. Med. *104* (1986) 455.

[47] Tormey, D. C., M. E. Lippman, B. K. Edwards et al.: Evaluation of Tamoxifen Doses with and without Fluoxymesterone in Advanced Breast Cancer. Ann. Intern. Med. *98* (1983) 139.

[48] Twito, D. I., J. N. Ingle, M. N. Chang et al.: Randomized Trial of Tamoxifen (TAM) alone of combined with Fluoxymesterone (FLU) in Postmenopausal Women with Metastatic Breast Cancer. ASCO 5 (1986) Abstr. 242, 62.

[49] van Veelen, H., P. H. B. Willemse, T. Tjabbes et al.: Oral High-Dose Medroxyprogesterone Acetate Versus Tamoxifen. Cancer *58* (1986) 7.

[50] Viladiu, P., M. C. Alonso, A. Avella et al.: Chemotherapy versus chemotherapy plus hormontherapy in postmenopausal advanced breast cancer patients. A randomized trial. Cancer *56* (1985) 2745.

[51] Wallgren, A., U. Glas, R. Buchanan et al.: A comparison of "nolvadex" (tamoxifen) monotherapy with "nolvadex" plus "halotestin" (fluoxymesterone) in the treatment of advanced breast cancer in postmenopausal women. Proc. 14th Int. Cancer Congr. (1986) Abstr. 4826.

[52] Westerberg, H.: Tamoxifen and Fluoxymesterone in Advanced Breast Cancer: A Controlled Clinical Trial. Cancer Treat. Rep. *64* (1980) 117.

State of the art in cytotoxic manipulation in treatment of metastatic breast cancer

I. C. Henderson

The present state of the art in the use of chemotherapy for the treatment of breast cancer might be summarized as: "many hypotheses, few experiments." The physician's ability to palliate metastatic breast cancer was markedly increased in the late 1950s when cytotoxic therapy was first used for this disease. From then until the mid-1970s increasingly more effective agents and combinations of drugs were added to the physician's armanentarium, and at one time it seemed as if "cure" of breast cancer was just around the corner. Unfortunately, however, rapid progress seems to have ended in the mid-1970s, and there is little evidence that new drugs introduced since then or innovations in the way we use these drugs has resulted in substantial improvement in either survival or quality of life for our patients.

This plateau in our progress is not from a lack of new ideas. The use of alternating non-cross resistant regimens, continuous infusion therapy, sequential methotrexate – 5-fluorouracil, a variety of sequences of hormonal therapy followed by chemotherapy, the combination of 5-fluorouracil and leucovorin, high dose therapy, and high dose-rate therapy all represent strategies based on sound scientific rationale. The data from small pilot trials provide promise that one or a combination of these approaches will substantially improve results. However, none has yet been shown in randomized trials to either significantly or substantially improve survival of patients with metastatic disease. However, their impact on patient quality of life may be slightly greater.

The hypothesis most extensively studied is that of alternating regimens, often times referred to as the Goldie – Coldman hypothesis. These investigators concluded from mathematical models that cancer patients develop resistance to chemotherapy programs very early after initiation of therapy, probably because of drug induced resistance in some cases. Goldie and Coldman hypothesized that the early introduction of a non-cross resistant regimen would result in a greater total tumor cell kill, and possibly cure even in some patients whose resistant tumor burden is small. This argument is compelling, and a series of randomized trials have been performed in patients with metastatic breast cancer to test the

Table 1 Randomized trials comparing a single regimen with alternating non-cross-resistant regimens [1]

Regimen (*)	No. of patients	Response rate (%) PR + CR	CR	Median duration (mos.) of Response	Survival	Reference
CFP vs.	23	48	15	12	24	
A/L-PAM vs.	27	52	9	13	21	
CFP → A/L-PAM or (2) A/L-PAM → CFP	50	68^{+}	10	16	22	388
CA vs.	26	50	12	10	–	390
CA ↔ MF (1)	22	55	32	10	–	
CAF vs.	46	63	13	–	–	
DAV ↔ CMF (3)	48	71	10	–	–	
CFP vs.	18	18	0	9	14	333
CA vs.	42	42	2	12	18	
CFP ↔ CA (1)	20	63^{++}	0	11	19	
CMF vs.	47	55	17	8	12	389
CMF ↔ AV (2)	50	58	22	12^{++}	18^{+++}	
CMFP vs.	135	59	14	11	19	389
CMFP ↔ AV (2)	176	58	14	10	16	
CAF vs.	66	29	2	8	15	391
CAF ↔ CAMELEON (3)	91	17^{+}	0	11	16	
CFP vs.	41	46	7	–	18	229
CAP → CFP (4)	45	49	4	–	11	

Abbreviations: C = Cyclophosphamide; A = doxorubicin; F = 5-fluorouracil; P = prednisone; L-PAM = L-phenylalanine mustard; M = methotrexate; D = dibromodulcitol (mitolactol); V = vincristine; T = tamoxifen; H = fluoxymesterone CAMELEON = cytosine arabinoside, methotrexate, leucovorin rescue, vincristine.
PR = partial response; CR = complete response

(*) Number of cycles before first crossover and/or number of cycles between each subsequent regimen alteration. + $p = 0.07-0.08$ ++ $p = 0.02-0.03$ +++ $p = 0.05$; other differences not statistically significant.

hypothesis (table 1) [1]. These trials have varied in size from about 50 patients to more than 300. However, the results are remarkably similar. In several of the studies there is a statistically significant increase in response rate, but in at least as many the response to an alternating regimen is the same or even slightly smaller than the response rate when only one of the two alternating regimens is used. A significant difference in survival was observed in only one of the studies, and even the duration of response was not markedly improved in most of them. One of the most interesting of these studies was that performed by the Mayo Clinic [2]. Patients were randomized to receive either CFP (cyclophosphamide, 5-fluorouracil, prednisone) or A/L-Pam (doxorubicin plus L-phenylalanine mustard). After two cycles of therapy patients on each of these combinations were randomized for crossover to the other. The overall response rate among patients crossed over was significantly higher (68%) than that among patients who continued on the original regimen (48% and 52%). However, the duration of response among patients crossed over was only marginally longer (16 months) compared to those continued on the same regimen (12 and 13 months), and the survival was not improved at all (22 months versus 21 and 24 months). The Eastern Cooperative Oncology Group (ECOG) randomized patients to receive either CMF (cyclophosphamide, methotrexate, and 5-fluorouracil) or CMF alternating with AV (doxorubicin plus vincristine) [3]. Interestingly, the response rate to the alternating program was not higher than that to the single regimen, but the duration of response and the duration of survival were significantly improved. Because of this seeming conflict, the ECOG repeated the trial with a larger number of patients, but in the second trial the comparison was made between CMFP (CMF plus prednisone) and CMFP alternating with AV. This alternating program did not prove to be superior in response rate, duration of response, or duration of survival, probably because CMFP is superior to CMF.

The cancer and leukemia group B (CALGB) designed a study to test the Goldie – Coldman hypothesis in the adjuvant setting [4]. Patients with histologically positive nodes were randomized to receive a six-month induction therapy with one of two doseschedules of CMFVP (CMF plus vincristine and prednisone). Thereafter patients were further randomized to continue on CMFVP or to cross over to VATH (vinblastine, doxorubicin, thiotepa, and halotestin). This trial was begun in October of 1980 and closed in August of 1984. Although 940 patients were accrued to the program (41% premenopausal), the results are still preliminary. However, at this time there is a highly significant disease-free survival advantage for those patients who received the cross over regimen, and survival differences are approaching statistical significance.

The results of the CALGB trial have not yet been confirmed by other investigators, and it is possible that when a series of trials are available to evaluate the Goldie – Coldman hypothesis in the adjuvant setting the results will be inconsistent. However, if the results of the CALGB trial are confirmed, this experience with the study of alternating regimens suggests principles that may be important in future breast cancer studies. One reason for contradictory results among trials in patients with metastatic disease may be the relatively small size of most of these trials. Chemotherapy trials among patients with metastases rarely exceed 200 patients, and it may require studies of the size of the CALGB trial to detect modest gains. If so, it is plausible that in the future our principles for the treatment of metastatic disease will be defined as much by the studies of early breast cancer, where large, definitive randomized trials are easily performed. This is in contrast to the more traditional approach of using the results of metastatic disease studies to justify adjuvant therapy investigations.

The list of new drugs introduced in the past decade is long and discouraging. Only a few have shown activity for breast cancer, and most of these have, as yet, failed to find a niche in the standard treatment of the disease (table 2) [1]. One of the most interesting of these agents is cisplatin. In a series of Phase II trials enrolling almost 100 patients, the overall response rate was a discouraging 8%. This was somewhat surprising in light of the high activity for cisplatin in a number of other tumors. However the patients in most of these phase II breast cancer studies had been heavily pretreated. Recently a single report on the activity of cisplatin in 20 previously untreated patients suggested that the response rate might be much higher [5]. Until now the major emphasis in new drug research has been on the discovery of non-cross resistant agents, in part because of wide spread conviction that the Goldie – Coldman hypothesis is a rate limiting step to further progress in the treatment of breast cancer. However, discovery of powerful but cross resistant agents provides at least an opening for the exploration of new therapeutic combinations and sequences not previously evaluated.

One of the most carefully evaluated of the new agents is mitoxantrone. In randomized trials comparing single agent mitoxantrone with single agent doxorubicin, there was a trend for a higher response rate among those patients given doxorubicin (table 3) [6]. However, in most of these studies this difference was

Table 2 Newer drugs for breast cancer (modified and updated from [1])

Drug	No. of patients studied	No prior chemo	Response rate (%) All patients	No prior chemo
Cisplatin	119	20	8	45
4'-Demethosydaunorubicin	121	57	26	37
4'-Deoxydoxorubicin	56	23	11	17
Elliptinium	228	66	27	37
4'-Epidoxorubicin	210	30	34	73
Mitolactol	142	0	17	–
Mitoxantrone	694	203	20	27
Vindesine	195	24	23	39

Table 3 Randomized trials of mitoxantrone

Single agent trials

Trial	Dose (mg/M²) of Mitox-antrone	Dose (mg/M²) of Doxo-rubicin	No. of patients	Response rate (%) Mitox-antrone	Response rate (%) Doxo-rubicin
Ohio	12	60	90 (24)	18	32
Lederle Co-op	14	75	325 (115)	20	29
SWOG	14	60	265 (56)	15	28*

* $p = 0.05$
( ) = Number without prior chemotherapy for metastases

Combination regimen trials

Trial	Study design	No. of patients	Response rate (%) Mitox-antrone	Response rate (%) Non-mitox-antrone
Lederle Co-op	CNF vs. CAF	331	29	37
Ottawa	CNF vs. CAF	–	–	–
Lima	NMF vs. CMF	35	72	65
Scotland	VNP vs. VAP	115	35	61*

* $p = 0.01$

not statistically significant. Mitroxantrone has also been included in a number of combination programs. While the combination NMF (mitoxantrone, methotrexate, and 5-fluorouracil) appears to be equal to that of CMF, this was not true when VMP (vincristine, mitoxantrone, and prednisone) was compared to VAP (vincristine, doxorubicin, and prednisone). CNF appears to be approximately equal to CAF in the largest of these trials.

While the activity of mitoxantrone appears to be equal or only slightly inferior to that of doxorubicin in these trials, the toxicity of mitoxantrone was substantially and statistically significantly less than that of doxorubicin. This was most evident when the alopecia induced by the two drugs was compared. Mitoxantrone causes mild alopecia in only about 20% of patients. Doxorubicin causes alopecia severe enough to require a wig in the majority of patients. Mitoxantrone also causes significantly less nausea, vomiting, and mucositis. This toxicity profile favoring mitoxantrone persisted even when it was used in combination with other drugs. Mitoxantrone is also less cardiotoxic when used either as a single agent or in combination. Finally, the survival of patients in most of these trials was identical regardless of the regimen received. One exception to this was the single agent study by SWOG (Southwest Oncology Group) where there was an overall survival advantage for the patients receiving doxorubicin, but this advantage was limited to those patients with a more aggressive form of the disease – i. e. those with a poor performance status, abnormal liver function tests, and a negative receptor status.

In general, the therapy of metastatic breast cancer has a marginal effect on patient survival. Patients randomized in trials to the less effective of two regimens almost always have the same survival as those randomized to the more effective (i. e. higher response rate) regimen. This has been true in most of the studies comparing a doxorubicin containing regimen with a combination of drugs without doxorubicin [7]. More recently this general observation has been confirmed in studies comparing high and low dose therapy and studies comparing continuous and intermittent chemotherapy. One of the earliest studies to show this was a Swiss trial in which patients were randomized to receive a combination of chemotherapy and hormonal therapy or hormonal therapy with a delay in the initiation of chemotherapy until evidence of progressive disease (or at least a lack of response to hormonal therapy) [8]. In this trial the response rate to patients given the chemo-endocrine therapy combination was significantly higher than the response to endocrine therapy alone. Survival of the two groups was nearly identical. However, there is a widely held opinion that the patients who benefit from “aggressive therapy” are those with the more “aggressive” forms of breast cancer. “Aggressive therapy” is often interpreted as meaning “early” chemotherapy. To address this issue the Swiss retrospectively stratified patients into high risk and low risk groups. There was no difference in the survival of premenopausal women randomized to the two study arms whether the patients were in the high risk or low risk categories. However, among postmenopausal women it was observed that there was a statistically significant survival disadvantage for postmenopausal women who were low risk and who were randomized to receive early chemotherapy. This suggests that under some circumstances, at least, aggressive therapy may in fact be harmful, and this may counterbalance those few studies that suggest there is a survival advantage for aggressive therapy in patients with aggressive disease.

In contrast to the effect of therapy on patient survival, the effect of therapy on the palliation of symptoms is often closely related to the efficacy of the therapy. It has repeatedly been shown that patients randomized to a regimen with a high response rate experience a better quality of life.

The first to illustrate this may have been Baum and Priestman in a study comparing patients randomized to receive either endocrine therapy or chemotherapy [9]. These investigators pioneered the use of a technique often referred to as LASA or Linear Analog Self-Assessment Evaluation. Patients taking this test are asked to indicate by placing a vertical tick along a horizontal line their relative feeling on a scale of 0 – 10. Thus patients will be asked to indicate whether they feel "lousy," feel "great," or somewhere between these two extremes. Other categories of response deal with pain, fatigue, dyspnea, anorexia, nausea/vomiting, irritability, apprehension, depression, sense of well being, insomnia, social relations, relations within the family, sexual functioning, and ability to do housework, regular employment, hobbies, or shopping. In the study by Baum et al. the response rate to chemotherapy was almost double that to endocrine therapy. The survival of patients on the two treatment arms was not significantly different. The side effects associated with the chemotherapy were significantly greater than with endocrine therapy. However, in spite of this the LASA scores for responders were higher than for non-responders, and in some categories the LASA scores were higher for patients given chemotherapy than endocrine therapy. It is plausible, then, that the higher response rate to chemotherapy resulted in a higher quality of life in spite of the greater toxicity associated with chemotherapy.

Two other trials have confirmed these results by Priestman and Baum. In a study performed by the Australian-New Zealand Breast Cancer Trials Group 307 patients were randomized to receive either continuous chemotherapy until evidence of disease progression or intermittent courses lasting no longer than three months with reinitiation of short course chemotherapy at the time of progression [10]. It was hypothesized prior to the initiation of this trial that the intermittent courses of chemotherapy would be associated with fewer cumulative side effects from therapy and thus a better quality of life. It was not surprising that the overall response rate to the continuous regimen was twice that seen with the intermittent regimen, but it was somewhat surprising that the quality of life (measured by LASA) among patients receiving the more toxic continuous chemotherapy was also significantly greater than the quality of life among those given the less toxic intermittent regimen. Tannock and his colleagues in Toronto have recently compared a standard intravenous dose of CMF chemotherapy with a low dose intravenous regimen [11]. The doses of the low dose program were exactly half those in the standard dose regimen, and the schedule of drug administration was the same in the two treatment arms. The response rate with standard dose CMF was nearly three times that achieved with the low dose regimen, and this difference was statistically significant. The survival advantage for patients on the high dose was marginal. As might be expected, there was a significantly higher incidence of nausea, vomiting, and hair loss among those patients given the standard dose program. However, there was also a significant improvement in a variety of non-treatment related parameters of quality of life (measured by LASA), including reduction of pain and anxiety and an increase in physical activity and social activity.

Patients enrolled on a randomized single agent trial comparing mitoxantrone and doxorubicin were also evaluated using the LASA technique [12]. As in these other studies, the quality of life for responders to either mitoxantrone or doxorubicin was significantly greater than that of the non-responders to either of the drugs. However, unlike the trials described above, the quality of life of patients treated with the lower response rate agent, mitoxantrone, was equal to or slightly superior to that of patients treated with doxorubicin. This mitoxantrone trial suggests balance between response rate and quality of life is delicate. In this instance, the palliative benefit from mitoxantrone appears to equal that of doxorubicin. This suggests that even though there is a higher response rate to doxorubicin, the lower response rate and lower toxicity associated with mitoxantrone therapy resulted in equal or slightly better quality of life.

A concept under intensive study at the present time is that of dose response [13]. Animal studies have repeatedly demonstrated that a small increment in drug dose may result in a disproportionately large increase in tumor cell kill. However, laboratory studies have also shown that this is a complex phenomenon dependent upon a large number of factors including the specific drug used, the intrinsic chemosensitivity of the tumor, the kinetic state of the tumor, tumor mass independent of the kinetic state, and the schedule of drug utilized. It cannot be assumed on the basis of the laboratory studies that there will be a dose response in the clinic, and these studies suggest that breast cancer is an unlikely tumor for a steep dose response curve.

Most of the studies of dose response have been retrospective analyses of randomized trials. One of the first to demonstrate the dose response was Bonadonna and his colleagues at the Milan Cancer Institute in Italy [14]. They were able to show that patients who received a higher cumulative dose of adjuvant CMF had improved disease free survival and overall survival compared to patients who had dose reductions for any reason. A large number of investigators have performed similar retrospective analyses of their trials, and approximately an equal number have confirmed and refuted the original hypothesis generated by the Milan group [13]. Pilot studies utilizing moderately high doses have also been interpreted as showing evidence of a dose response. These include a trial of "Super-CMF" performed at the Dana Farber Cancer Institute [15], a trial of "DAV-MP-HxTHBleo" studied at the University of Wisconsin [16], and a high dose combination of cyclophosphamide and 5-fluorouracil evaluated by L. Israel in France [17].

One of the most frequently cited analyses of dose is that by Hryniuk from Hamilton, Ontario [18, 19]. This is actually a comparison of chemotherapy dose-rate and outcome in a number of unrelated trials. The report of dose-rate in adjuvant chemotherapy studies includes study arms in which no therapy was given, regimens utilizing L-phenylalanine mustard alone or in combination, and a variety of CMF $\pm$ VP regimens. This analysis assumes a fixed relationship between the dose of L-phenylalanine mustard and cyclophosphamide that has not been demonstrated in clinical trials. Furthermore, it assumes that the effect of any two drugs at half-dose is identical to that of one drug at full dose. In other words, this analysis rejects the possibility of drug synergy or a differential sensitivity to drugs among different clones of tumor cells. Hryniuk observed a highly significant relationship between dose and three year disease free survival for all treated patients, for all nodal subgroups, and for patients in all menopausal groups [19]. However, this has been re-analyzed by Gelman and Henderson [20] (table 4). The re-analysis is limited to trials in which CMF is included and excludes the arms with no adjuvant therapy and those that utilized L-phenylalanine mustard. As a result, the re-analysis avoids some of the major assumptions required by the Hyrniuk analysis. However, in the re-analysis there was no evidence for a dose-rate effect. In fact, the correlation coefficient for premenopausal women was negative, implying that a higher dose rate was associated with a poorer three year relapse-free survival.

Results from randomized trials evaluating dose are more limited but suggest, in contrast to the conclusions from small pilot studies and retrospective analyses, that the importance of dose is less certain. The Canadian dose study, described above, is the only randomized study comparing standard doses of therapy with reduced doses [11]. As summarized, the higher doses were associated with a higher response rate, a marginal improvement in survival, a significant increase in toxicity, and a significant increase in the quality of life. The definitive

Table 4 Regression analysis of disease-free survival on dose intensity of adjuvant chemotherapy [13]

Treatment group	Correlation coefficient (r) Hryniuk* [19]	Correlation coefficient (r) Reanalysis** [20]	p-Value Hryniuk* [19]	p-Value Reanalysis** [20]
All patients	0.81	0.13	<0.00001	0.69
Premenopausal				
1–3 positive nodes	0.52	−0.40	0.001	0.14
>4 positive nodes	0.57	−0.02	<0.001	0.94
Postmenopausal				
1–3 positive nodes	0.54	0.12	0.002	0.72
>4 positive nodes	0.56	0.05	0.002	0.89

A positive correlation (coefficient r) suggests that 3 year disease-free survival increased as dose intensity increased.

* Studies included those with no chemotherapy, melphalan alone, cyclophosphamide alone, melphalan + fluorouracil, melphalan + MF, CMF, CMFV, CMFP, and CMFVP.

** Limited to studies of CMF, CMFV, CMFP, and CMFVP.

randomized trial comparing standard dose chemotherapy with high dose chemotherapy is from M. D. Anderson [21]. In this study a standard dose of FAC (5-fluorouracil, doxorubicin, cyclophosphamide) was compared to maximally tolerated doses of the same regimen. The randomization applied only to the induction therapy. However, no significant difference in response rate, time to response, median duration of response, or survival was observed. Two studies not specifically designed to evaluate dose have inadvertently done so. In one of these trials, Ludwig I, patients were randomized to receive either adjuvant CMF or CMFP [22]. Because the prednisone in the CMFP regimen (CMF plus continuous prednisone) resulted in less myelosuppression, the patients on the CMFP received a higher total dose of drug. Nonetheless, there was no significant difference in disease free survival or overall survival for patients receiving CMFP. In the CALGB adjuvant trial of alternating regimens, described above, patients inadvertently received two different dose-rates of CMFVP during the induction phase of therapy [23]. However, patients receiving the more intensive dose-rate of CMFVP did not have an improvement in prolongation of either time to recurrence or overall survival. The CALGB is currently performing a randomized trial comparing three different doses of adjuvant CAF, but results from this trial will not be available for some years yet.

In trials described thus far, myelosuppression has served as the dose-limiting factor. However, recent technology permits circumvention of this dose limitation by the use of either colony-stimulating factors or autologous bone marrow transplantation. The data utilizing CSF is still too limited to provide any meaningful analysis at the present time. However, almost 250 patients have been studied in a large number of small trials utilizing very high doses of chemotherapy, usually an alkylating agent, with autologous bone marrow support [13]. In many of these trials the overall response rate was high, approaching 100% in some instances, but overall about 50% of the patients have responded and about 25% have had a complete response. Most of the patients entered on to these studies had no further treatment after one course of high dose chemotherapy with re-infusion of bone marrow, and this may explain the relatively short median duration of response and survival in most of these studies. As might be expected, toxicity observed in these studies is unusually high in spite of the use of bone marrow re-infusion. Overall the toxic mortality is about 10%, but in individual studies this reaches levels of 20–35%. A strategy currently being employed at many centers is the use of high dose therapy and autologous marrow support as an "adjuvant" after induction of a partial or complete response with conventional dose therapy. One of the earliest trials to study this concept was that of the Royal Marsden in London. These patients were given high doses of L-phenylalanine mustard following induction and response. Patients were then retrospectively matched with similar patients treated in the same clinic who had not received high dose therapy and bone marrow transplantation. Investigators at the Royal Marsden concluded from this historically controlled study that survival was not prolonged.

The available data suggest that dose should not be decreased below standard levels for trivial reasons, but there is little evidence that reduced doses significantly compromise patient survival in either the metastatic or adjuvant setting. At present there are insufficient data to justify increasing doses above standard levels in routine practice, but high dose therapy with CSF or autologous marrow support should be tested in randomized trials.

Overall conclusions

The major value of chemotherapy in the treatment of patients with metastatic disease is palliation. Survival is, on average, only marginally prolonged. Regimens associated with a higher response rate are usually associated with an improvement in overall quality of life. In most, but not all, instances the higher response rate is associated with improved quality of life in spite of increased toxicity. At the present time the point at which additional toxicity outweighs additional benefit is not well defined in most clinical settings.

Higher response rates are usually obtained from combination chemotherapy rather than the use of single agents, for the use of combinations that include doxorubicin, from treatment duration in excess of three months, and possibly for the use of higher doses of therapy. However, it is still not clear that there is any improvement in survival from the use of drugs other than cyclophosphamide, methotrexate, 5-fluorouracil, doxorubicin and mitoxantrone. No substantial advantage has yet been reproducably demonstrated for the use of alternating regimens. Although more than three months of therapy is beneficial, it is not yet clear that continuous therapy until disease progression is superior to more limited durations. The use of continuous infusion therapy, sequential methotrexate/5-fluorouracil, and 5-fluorouracil + leucovorin remain to be carefully studied in randomized trials.

It seems likely that future progress in the treatment of metastatic breast cancer will be achieved by combining small to moderate benefits from several different strategies. Since an increase in response rate is rarely associated with an increase in survival, other endpoints that better reflect total tumor cell kill need to be evaluated. Possibly time to treatment failure will prove to be a practical endpoint of this type. Many of the strategies currently under evaluation are aimed at improvement in the survival of patients with "aggressive tumors." However, these tumors constitute a small proportion of all patients with early or advanced breast cancer. Future strategies should place equal emphasis on the treatment of multiple tumor clones, especially cell clones characterized by a low growth fraction.

References

[1] Henderson, I. C.: Chemotherapy for Advanced Disease. In: J. R. Harris, S. Hellman, I. C. Henderson et al. (eds.): Breast Diseases. Lippincott, Co., Philadelphia 1987.

[2] Ahmann, D., J. O'Fallon, M. T. O'Connell et al.: Evaluation of a Fixed Alternating Treatment in Patients with Advanced Breast Cancer. Cancer Clin. Trials *1* (1978) 219 – 226.

[3] Tormey, D., R. Gelman, G. Falkson: Prospective Evaluation of Rotating Chemotherapy in Advanced Breast Cancer. Am. J. Clin. Oncol. *6* (1983) 1 – 18.

[4] Perloff, M., L. Norton, A. Korzun et al.: Advantage of an Adriamycin (A) Combination Plus Halotestin (H) After Initial Cyclophosphamide, Methotrexate, 5-Fluorouracil, Vincristine and Prednisone (CMFP) for Adjuvant Therapy of Node-Positive Stage II Breast Cancer. Proc. Am. Soc. Clin. Oncol. *5* (1986) 70.

[5] Sledge, Jr., G. W., P. J. Loehrer, Sr., B. J. Roth et al.: Cisplatin as First-Line Therapy for Metastatic Breast Cancer. Proc. Am. Soc. Clin. Oncol. *6* (1987) 53.

[6] Henderson, I. C.: Mitoxantrone for Advanced Breast Cancer: Comparison with Other Standard Agents. In: H. T. Mouridsen, Z. A. Arlin (eds.): Pharmamanual. PharmaLibri, Chicago 1987.

[7] Henderson, I. C.: The Meaning of a Response in Patients with Metastatic Breast Cancer. In: C. G. Schmidt, K. W. Brunner, E. Enghofer (eds.): Therapiestrategien beim metastasierten Mammakarzinom. De Gruyter, Berlin – New York 1987.

[8] Cavalli, F., M. Beer, G. Martz et al.: Concurrent or Sequential Use of Cytotoxic Chemotherapy and Hormone Treatment. In: Advanced Breast Cancer: Report of the Swiss Group for Clinical Cancer Research. Br. Med. J. *286* (1983) 5 – 8.

[9] Baum, M., T. Priestman, R. R. West et al.: A Comparison of Subjective Responses in a Trial Comparing Endocrine with Cytotoxic Treatment in Advanced Carcinoma of the Breast. In: H. T. Mouridsen, T. Palshof (eds.): Breast Cancer – Experimental and Clinical Aspects. Pergamon Press, Oxford 1980.

[10] Coates, A., V. Gebski, J. F. Bishop et al.: Improving the Quality of Life During Chemotherapy for Advanced Breast Cancer. New Engl. J. Med. *317* (1987) 1490 – 1495.

[11] Tannock, I. F., N. F. Boyd, G. DeBoer et al.: A Randomized Trial of Two Dose Levels of CMF Chemotherapy for Patients with Metastatic Breast Cancer. J. Clin. Oncol. *20* (1988) (In Press.)

[12] Henderson, I. C., S. Wolff, J. Allegra et al.: A Randomized Trial Comparing Mitoxantrone and Doxorubicin in Patients with Metastatic Breast Cancer. In: C. A. Coltman Jr. (ed.): The Current Status of Novantrone. John Wiley and Sons, New York 1985.

[13] Henderson, I. C., D. F. Hayes, R. Gelman: Dose Response in the Treatment of Breast Cancer: A Critical Review. J. Clin. Oncol. (1988) (In Press.)

[14] Bonadonna, G., P. Valagussa, A. Rossi et al.: Ten-Year Experience with CMF-Based Adjuvant Chemotherapy in Resectable Breast Cancer. Breast Cancer Res. Treat. 5 (1985) 95 – 115.

[15] Henderson, I. C., R. Gelman, G. P. Canellos et al.: III. Prolonged Disease-Free Survival in Advanced Breast Cancer Treated With "Super-CMF" Adriamycin: An Alternating Regimen Employing High-Dose Methotrexate with Citrovorum Factor Rescue. Cancer Treat. Rep. 65 (1981) 67 – 75.

[16] Tormey, D. C., J. C. Kline, M. Palta et al.: Short Term High Density Systemic Therapy for Metastatic Breast Cancer. Breast Cancer Res. Treat. 5 (1985) 177 – 188.

[17] Israel, L., J. L. Breau, J. Aguilera: High-Dose Cyclosphosphamide and High-Dose 5-Fluorouracil: A New First-Line Regimen for Advanced Breast Cancer. Cancer 53 (1984) 1655 – 1659.

[18] Hryniuk, W., H. Bush: The Importance of Dose Intensity in Chemotherapy of Metastatic Breast Cancer. J. Clin. Oncol. 2 (1984) 1281 – 1288.

[19] Hryniuk, W., M. N. Levine: Analysis of Dose Intensity for Adjuvant Chemotherapy Trials in Stage II Breast Cancer. J. Clin. Oncol. 4 (1986) 1162 – 1170.

[20] Gelman, R. S., I. C. Henderson: A Reanalysis of Dose Intensity for Adjuvant Chemotherapy Trials in Stage II Breast Cancer. SAKK Bulletin *1* (1987) 10 – 12.

[21] Hortobagyi, G. N., A. U. Buzdar, G. P. Bodey et al.: High-Dose Induction Chemotherapy of Metastatic Breast Cancer in Protected Environment: A Prospective Randomized Study. J. Clin. Oncol. 5 (1987) 178 – 184.

[22] Ludwig Breast Cancer Study Group: A Randomized Trial of Adjuvant Combination Chemotherapy With or Without Prednisone in Premenopausal Breast Cancer Patients with Metastases in one to three Axillary Lymph Nodes. Cancer Res. 45 (1985) 4454 – 4459.

[23] Korzun, A., L. Norton, M. Perloff et al.: Clinical Equivalence Despite Dosage Differences of Two Schedules of Cyclophosphamide, Methotrexate, 5-Fluorouracil, Vincristine, and Prednisone (CMFVP) for Adjuvant Therapy of Node-Positive Stage II Breast Cancer. Proc. Am. Soc. Clin. Oncol. 7 (1988) 12.

[24] Vincent, M. D., T. J. Powles, R. C. Coombes et al.: Late Intensification with High Dose Melphalan and Autologous Bone Marrow Support in Breast Cancer Patients Responding to Conventional Chemotherapy. Cancer Chemother. Pharmacol. (1988) (In Press.)

New aspects of the diagnosis and treatment of breast cancer

R. C. Coombes, R. C. Stein

The Clinical Oncology Unit at St George's Hospital is involved in research in the basic biology and in clinical management of breast cancer. We describe in this paper some of our work on the applications of monoclonal and polyclonal antibody technology to aspects of diagnosis and on the development of new drugs for the treatment of breast cancer.

Oestrogen receptors

Approximately 60% of breast cancers are classified as being positive for oestrogen receptor (ER). Conventionally ER is assayed using biochemical techniques; the dextran coated charcoal (DCC) assay [26] is the most widely used method of ER determination. It is usual to classify tumours as being ER positive if more than 10 – 15 fmol of oestrogen binding per milligram of cytosol protein is detected. This cut off, which has been set arbitrarily, predicts a probability of response to endocrine treatment of approximately 50%. Unfortunately 300 – 500 mg of tissue are required for the DCC assay, necessitating a formal surgical biopsy and preventing determination of ER status when only small amounts of tissue are available.

Using immunocytochemical techniques it is now possible to detect ER in individual cells [23, 24]. The technique uses a monoclonal antibody directed against the ER which is visualised using an alkaline phosphatase conjugate. There is an excellent correlation between the proportion of cells staining for ER and the ER content of tumours as determined by DCC assay (fig. 1) ($r = 0.75$; $p < 0.001$) [25]. We have examined staining for ER prospectively in the tumours of 56 patients who subsequently received endocrine therapy for advanced disease. 22 patients had objectively documented responses to therapy and in 21 of these patients, >50% of tumour cells stained for ER. 8 out of the 34 non-responders had >50% staining for ER; 14 of the non-responders were ER positive by conventional DCC assay performed simultaneously. It is possible that immunocytochemical determination of ER status may prove to be a more sensitive and specific predictior of response to endocrine therapy than the DCC assay.

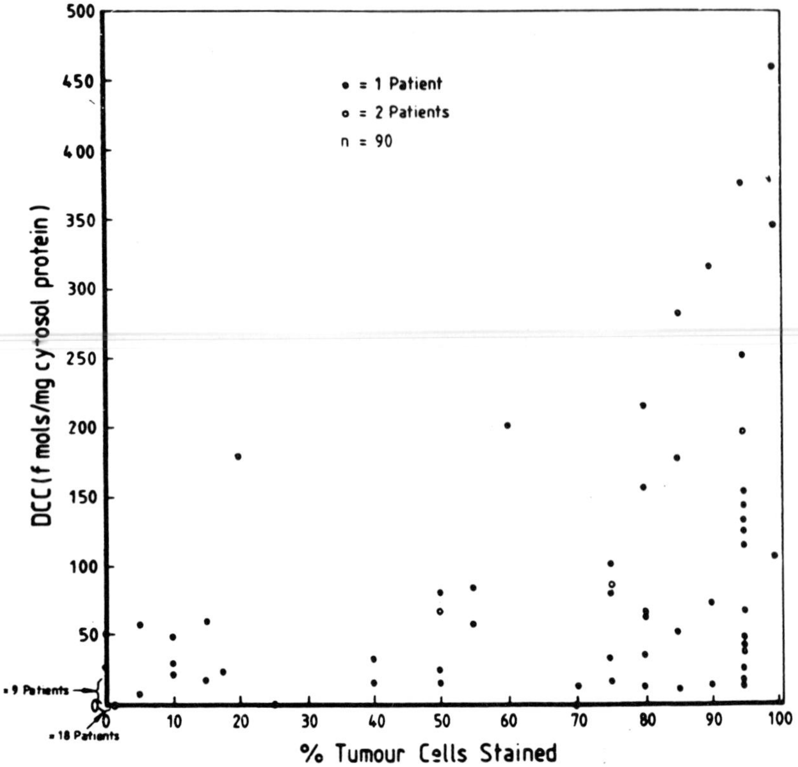

Fig. 1 Relationship between percentage of tumour cells stained by ERICA and DCC method.
$\pi = 0.75$ $p < 0.001$

Fine needle aspiration cytology in many cases is a satisfactory alternative for diagnostic purposes to formal surgical biopsy and histological examination. In breast cancer, the technique is of particular value in locally advanced and metastatic disease, in which surgery plays a relatively minor management role. We have extended the application of fine needle aspiration cytology to immunocytochemical determination of ER [6].

We have examined cytological specimens obtained from 60 patients with either locally advanced (11 patients) or metastatic disease (49 patients). Aspirates were taken from lymph nodes (11 patients), breast tumour (14 patients), skin nodules (25 patients) or locally recurrent cancers (10 patients). In 30 patients, aspirates were taken before any systemic therapy had been given; the remaining 30 patients had relapsed on first-line therapy and aspirates were taken before second-line treatment was initiated.

Aspirated material was smeared onto poly-L-lysine coated glass slides and frozen in dry ice or liquid nitrogen within 30 seconds, prior to fixation in 3.6% formol/

phosphate buffered saline followed by staining with an ER monoclonal antibody as previously described [6, 24]. A mirror image smear on a plain glass slide was prepared with each coated slide for cytology. This allowed examination of each specimen to ensure that there were adequate numbers of carcinoma cells present.

45 (75%) of 60 aspirates were considered adequate for evaluation of ER staining. The results classified according to the response of the patient to subsequent endocrine treatment are displayed in figure 2. 30 of the 45 samples contained cells that were positive for ER (20 – 100% of stained cells). 19 of the 21 patients who responded to subsequent endocrine treatment had smears which contained ER positive cells in contrast to 7 of the 18 non-responders ($p<0.001$). The mean percentage ($\pm$ SEM) of positive cells in responding patients was $58 \pm 6.1\%$ in contrast to $21 \pm 5.5\%$ in non-responding patients ($p<0.001$). 4 patients had 2 samples taken; the results were consistent in all 4 patients. Similarly 5 patients with ER positive aspirates also had ER immunocytochemistry positive biopsies.

Our results show that ER immunocytochemistry of fine needle aspirates is as useful a predictor of endocrine response as the DCC assay performed on biopsy

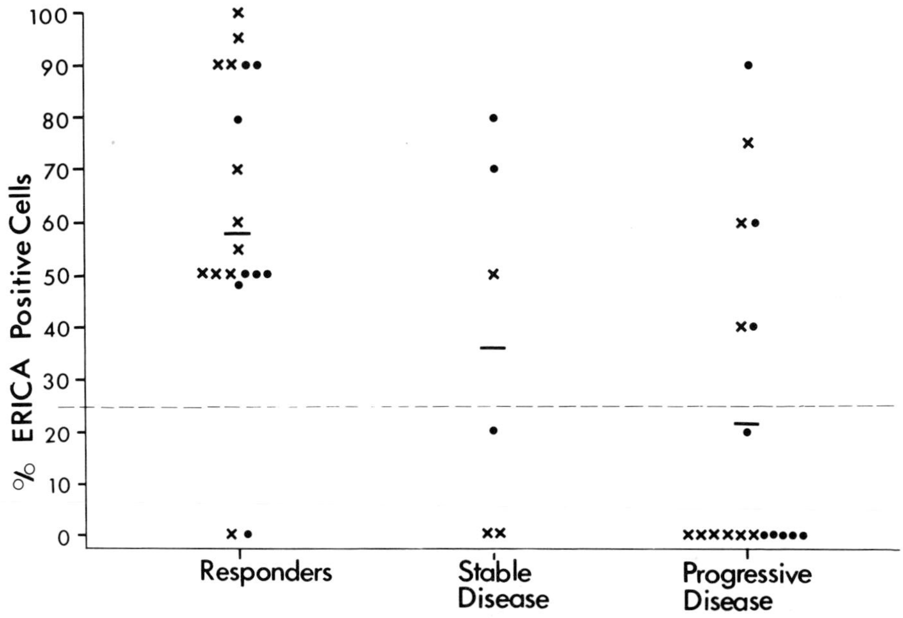

Fig. 2 Proportion of ER positive cells in samples from patients who received endocrine therapy.
X = sample obtained before first-line endocrine therapy
O = sample obtained before second-line therapy
Bars indicate means

specimens. We are currently investigating the potential of simultaneous progesterone receptor immunocytochemistry to improve the predictive value of ER immunocytochemistry.

The significance of micrometastases in primary breast cancer

The proportion of patients presenting with primary breast cancer with no evidence of distant metastases on conventional staging who relapse and die within 5 years is approximately 40%. It is widely believed that in the majority of these cases, the disease is disseminated at presentation but conventional imaging techniques are insufficiently sensitive to detect micrometastases. It is useful to be able to identify poor prognosis subgroups of patients; such patients may benefit from more intensive forms of systemic adjuvant therapy than are appropriate for patients with a better prognosis. At present a variety of indirect indices are used to predict the presence of occult metastatic disease (and hence prognosis). These include tumour size, histological grade and the presence or absence of vascular invasion, and the number of involved axillary lymph nodes.

We have attempted to use direct methods to detect the presence of occult micrometastases in patients with apparently localised primary breast cancer by examining bone marrow aspirates taken at the time of tumour resection. We have chosen bone marrow because the tissue is easy to obtain and because a high proportion of patients who relapse develop metastases in the axial skeleton [5, 21].

It is difficult to detect micrometastases in bone marrow using conventional haematological stains [7, 20, 31]. We have used an antiserum to epithelial membrane antigen raised in rabbit against human milk fat globule membranes [19, 28] which stains epithelial cells but not haemopoietic, lymphoid and connective tissue cells found in normal bone marrow [10–12, 32]. (We used a polyclonal antibody because at the time our study was initiated there was no readily available suitable monoclonal antibody.)

With the aid of the antibody we have screened bone marrow aspirates taken from 6 sites in 307 patients [10, 11, 27]. Tumour cells were detected in 81 (26.4%) patients. In none of 200 aspirates, which were stained using conventional techniques, were tumour cells detected. We have related the presence of micrometastases to various prognostic features. The data are shown in table 1. There was a significant association between the presence of tumour cells in the bone marrow and T stage, pathological size of tumour, presence of involved axillary nodes and vascular invasion, but not oestrogen receptor status or menopausal state. The actual number of cells detected in bone marrow showed no relation to any of the indirect prognostic indices. The vast majority of patients had infiltrating

Table 1 Clinical and pathological characteristics of patients

	Total	Micro-metastases: present number (%)		Micro-metastases: absent number (%)		Significance: degrees of freedom
T Stage						
T_0-T_2	222	44	(20)	178	(80)	$X^2 = 15.6$, df = 1
T_3-T_4	84	36	(43)	48	(57)	$p<0.001$
Pathological size (cm)						
<2	100	15	(15)	85	(85)	$p = 0.006$
2–5	173	57	(33)	116	(67)	X^2 (trend) = 7.54,
>5	12	3	(25)	9	(75)	df = 1
Nodal status						
− ve	152	29	(19)	123	(81)	$X^2 = 6.19$, df = 1
+ ve	135	44	(33)	91	(67)	$p = 0.013$
Not done	20	8		12		
Vascular invasion						
not seen	191	32	(17)	159	(83)	$X^2 = 22.8$, df = 1
+ ve	116	49	(42)	67	(58)	$p<0.001$
Oestrogen receptor						
− ve	92	31	(34)	61	(66)	$X^2 = 2.45$, df = 1
+ ve	199	48	(24)	151	(76)	$p = 0.12$
Not done	16	2		14		
Menopausal status						
pre-	77	20	(26)	57	(74)	$X^2 = 0.000$, df = 1
post-	230	61	(27)	169	(73)	$p = 0.96$

This table demonstrates the relation of various clinical and pathological characteristics of the patients to the presence or absence of tumour cells in the bone marrow at the time of primary surgery.

ductal carcinomas; the number of patients with the rarer subtypes including lobular carcinoma was too small to determine any relation to the presence of micrometastases.

Patients have been followed up for a median period of 28 months; 75 patients have relapsed, 60 of whom developed distant metastases. Of the patients developing distant metastases, 26 belonged to the group of 81 patients (32%) in whom micrometastases had been detected, whilst only 15% of the patients without tumour cells detected in bone marrow developed distant disease. The disease free

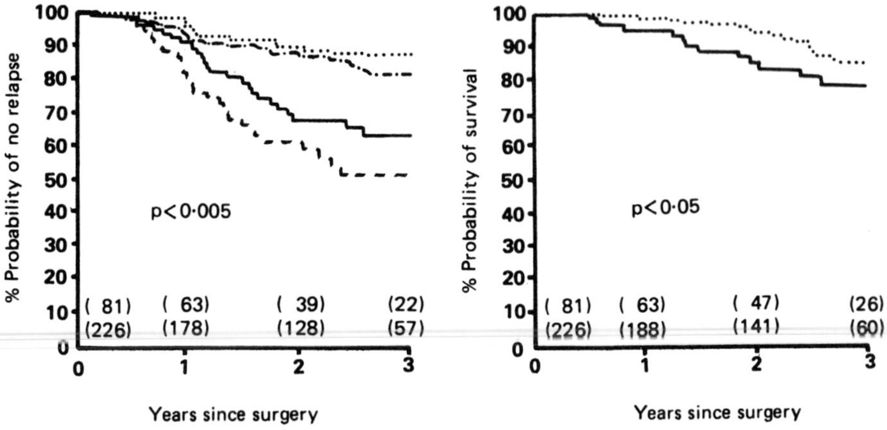

Fig. 3 (a) Disease-free survival according to the presence or absence of micrometastases at the time of initial surgery (left panel), and
(b) Overall survival (right panel)
Relapse at all sites i. e. local and distant is represented by .-.-.- EMA-negative, --- EMA-positive; relapse at distant sites only is represented by ... EMA-negative, — EMA-positive.
The number of patients at risk are shown along the x-axis.

interval and duration of survival were significantly worse in patients with micrometastases detected at the time of primary surgery (fig. 3).

19 patients developing distant metastases relapsed in bone, of whom 10 (53%) had micrometastases in comparison to 41 of the remaining 288 patients who remained disease free or relapsed at other sites. The predictive effect of the presence of tumour cells in bone marrow on the time to subsequent development of bone metastases was highly significant ($p<0.005$).

A Cox multivariate regression analysis has been performed to investigate whether the presence of micrometastases in bone marrow predicts relapse independently of other prognostic indicators. Pathological size was the most important prognostic indicator and lymph node involvement was also significant; both the presence of vascular invasion and micrometastases had a small positive effect but neither was independently significant (table 2). The Cox analysis for relapse in bone alone was qualitatively similar to the analysis for relapse in all sites.

Although we have failed to demonstrate that the presence of micrometastases in bone marrow is an independent prognostic indicator, there is clearly a relationship between micrometastases and relapse, especially with metastases in bone. It is possible that the sensitivity of our method could be improved by the use of a cocktail of antibodies rather than a single antibody; we are investigating such techniques.

Table 2 Cox regression analysis of time to first metastasis

Factor	Baseline	level	Co-efficient	Standard error	Hazard ratio	(95% Confidence interval)
a) All distant relapses						
Pathological size	<2 cm	2–5 cm	1.00	0.48	2.71	(1.06, 6.96)
	<2 cm	>5 cm	1.45	0.46	4.26	(1.73, 10.5)
Lymph. nodes	– ve	+ ve	0.66	0.32	1.92	(1.03, 3.62)
Vascular invasion	absent	present	0.50	0.32	1.65	(0.88, 3.09)
Micrometastases	absent	present	0.31	0.30	1.36	(0.76, 2.45)
b) Bone relapse only						
Pathological size	<2 cm	2–5 cm	0.36	0.74	1.43	(0.34, 6.11)
	<2 cm	>5 cm	1.15	0.66	3.17	(0.87, 11.5)
Lymph. nodes	– ve	+ ve	0.35	0.53	1.42	(0.50, 4.0)
Vascular invasion	absent	present	0.90	0.55	2.46	(0.84, 7.23)
Micrometastases	absent	present	0.81	0.50	2.24	(0.84, 5.99)

The independent effect of each factor on relapse free survival is assessed by modelling the effect at different levels of the factor compared to a baseline level. The coefficients obtained and the hazard ratio are given in the table. The hazard ratio estimates the ratio of the relapse rate in patients with the given level of the factor to the relapse in patients with the baseline level.

The ability to detect micrometastatic disease and its prognostic significance means that it is possible to monitor the course of disease and the effects of systemic adjuvant therapy in appropriate subgroups of patients who have not developed overt metastatic disease by performing serial bone marrow aspirates. We are currently undertaking such studies.

4-hydroxyandrostenedione in advanced breast cancer

We have conducted studies over the past ten years to obtain an optimal inhibitor of aromatase. Aminoglutethimide, whilst inducing remissions in patients with breast cancer, is suboptimal because (a) it causes significant side-effects, (b) it does not completely inhibit aromatase and (c) it inhibits the desmolase enzyme system requiring the co-administration of corticosteroids. (For reviews of its application in advanced breast cancer see [17] and in the adjuvant setting [8].)

4-hydroxyandrostenedione (4OHA) is a potent inhibitor of aromatase with no other known clinically significant pharmacological action at therapeutic doses.

In *in vitro* systems, it has been shown to have 60-fold greater activity than aminoglutethimide as an inhibitor of placental aromatase [2, 3]. 4OHA shows behaviour that is characteristic of a suicide inhibitor which irreversibly inactivates an enzyme by an attack on its active site, which is dependent upon the enzyme's own mechanism of action.

4OHA has been shown to be effective in causing tumour regression in the rat DMBA induced mammary carcinoma model. The preclinical studies of 4OHA have been summarised by Brodie et al [4].

Following the success of 4OHA in the animal model, we performed a pilot study in 11 previously treated postmenopausal women with advanced breast cancer, who received 500 mg of 4OHA by once weekly intramuscular injection [6]. Sustained falls in plasma oestradiol were recorded in all patients in whom measurements were made and in 4 patients there was objective evidence of tumour regression. We have subsequently performed 3 phase II studies of 4OHA treatment in breast cancer; these studies are described below.

All patients treated had histologically or cytologically proven locally advanced or metastatic breast cancer. Patients were either postmenopausal or had undergone oophorectomy at least one year before entry and had discontinued previous treatments 4 or more weeks before entry. 4OHA was given in doses of 500 mg by weekly intramuscular injection (group 1: [16]), 250 mg by alternate weekly intramuscular injection (group 2: [34]) or 500 mg daily by mouth, (group 3: [9]). The number of patients assessable for response was 131; a further 22 patients were evaluated for 4OHA toxicity although response assessments could not be made either because less than 3 weeks treatment was given or because disease was not assessable for response. The 3 studies, which were performed sequentially are summarised in table 3 and the characteristics of the patients assessable for response are shown in table 4. The characteristics of the non-assessable patients

Table 3 4-hydroxyandrostenedione treatment groups

Group	Dose	Route	Frequency	Number of patients Assessable for toxicity	 Assessable for response
1	500 mg	im	weekly	65	52
2	250 mg	im	2 weekly	57	55
3	500 mg	o	daily	31	24

Not assessable for response:

<3/52 treatment	13 (5 withdrawn for toxicity)
lost to followup	4
unassessable disease	5

Table 4 Characteristics of evaluable patients

	Group 1	Group 2	Group 3
Age Range	38 – 87	38 – 86	35 – 82
Median age	64	65	67
Number of prior endocrine treatments			
0	11	19	4
1	12	30	12
2	18	5	6
2 +	11	1	2
Prior endocrine response	26	21	17
Oestrogen receptor status			
positive	20	20	8
negative	4	5	5
unknown	28	30	11

did not differ significantly from those of the assessable patients. Patients in group 1, which was the first study to be performed, were more heavily pretreated than the patients entered in the later studies; the characteristics of the patients in the 3 studies were otherwise very similar.

4OHA was provided in the form of a sterile microcrystalline powder in ampoules (Ciba Geigy Pharmaceuticals CGP-32349); it was stored at 4° C until immediately prior to use when it was suspended in physiological saline at a concentration of 125 mg/ml. Parenteral administration was by deep intramuscular injection into the buttock. Injection sites were varied to improve local tolerability.

Patients were fully staged according to standard protocols prior to treatment, at intervals during treatment and on suspicion of progression. Response assessment was made according to UICC criteria [18]. Our methodology is fully described in the original reports [6, 13, 16].

Clinical results

A total of 131 patients were assessed for response. The overall results of treatment are shown in table 5. There were a total of 43 (33%) patients in whom an objective tumour regression occurred in at least one site as a result of 4OHA treatment, including 5 patients with a complete response. Disease stabilisation occurred in a further 19 (14%) patients. In 69 patients, disease progressed despite treatment. When the response data for the 3 studies are considered separately, the results of treatment in the 3 groups are extremely similar. No improvement in response status was achieved by increasing the dose of 4OHA to 1 g weekly

Table 5 Overall response to 4OHA

	Number of patients	Number (percentage) responding CR/PR		NC		PD	
Group 1	52	17	(33)	7	(13)	28	(54)
Group 2	55	18	(33)	8	(14)	29	(53)
Group 3	24	8	(33)	4	(17)	12	(50)
Total	131	43	(33)	19	(14)	69	(53)

CR = complete response PR = partial response
NC = no change PD = progressive disease

Table 6 Response according to oestrogen receptor status

	Number of patients	Number responding to 4OHA CR/PR	NC	PD
ER positive	48	14	7	27
ER negative	14	3	1	10
ER unknown	69	25	11	33

in 6 patients in group 1, and to 500 mg 2 weekly in 8 patients in group 2. One patient in group 1 whose dose of 4OHA was increased to 1 g weekly 3 months after commencement showed radiographic evidence of recalcification of bone lesions after 6 months of treatment; the significance of this in relation to the dose change in uncertain. Dose reductions were made in 9 patients in the 2 parenteral studies without apparent detriment.

The response to treatment according to oestrogen receptor status is shown in table 6. 3 patients with oestrogen receptor negative tumours responded to 4OHA treatment. All 3 patients had received previous endocrine treatment of whom 2 had responded; the 3rd was not assessable for response.

The results of 4OHA treatment according to previous endocrine treatment are shown in table 7. Of the 33 previously untreated patients in the 3 studies, there were 9 (27%) cases of tumour regression and 5 (15%) cases of stabilisation in response to 4OHA treatment. Of the 98 patients who had received one or more endocrine treatments prior to receiving 4OHA, 64 had responded. 29 of the 34 pretreated patients responding to 4OHA had responded to previous endocrine treatment. No patient responded to 4OHA who had progressed on all previous therapy.

Table 7 Response according to previous endocrine treatment

Previous endocrine treatment	Number of patients	Number responding to 4OHA CR/PR	NC	PD
None	33	9	5	19
Oophorectomy				
CR/PR	10	7	1	2
NC/PD	0			
Tamoxifen*				
CR/PR	53	22	10	21
NC/PD	18	3	1	14
Aminoglutethimide				
CR/PR	7	2	0	5
NC/PD	7	1	1	5
Medroxyprogesterone acetate				
CR/PR	5	1	0	4
NC/PD	7	1	1	5
Best overall response				
CR/PR	64	29	10	25
NC	6	3	1	2
PD	14	0	1	13
not assessable	14	2	3	9

* Includes 9 patients treated with combination of tamoxifen, aminoglutethimide and danazol.

Also shown in table 7 are the responses to 4OHA in terms of the outcome of previous endocrine treatment with individual agents. In addition to oophorectomy, tamoxifen, aminoglutethimide, and medroxyprogesterone acetate and a combination of tamoxifen, aminoglutethimide and danazol, a few patients were treated with danazol, decadurabolin and norethisterone acetate; these data are not shown in the table.

When response to 4OHA treatment is analysed according to disease site, the most favourable results were seen in patients with soft tissue disease, 38% of whom responded. The response rate in patients with involvement of the lung parenchyma was 19%, whilst 17% of patients with bone metastases showed radiographic evidence of healing. One of 18 patients with liver metastases responded at that site. The data are summarised in table 8.

The median duration of progression free treatment in responding patients was 10 months in group 1 and 12 months in group 2. The data are not available for group 3.

Table 8 Response according to disease site

Site	Number of patients	Number (percentage) responding
Soft tissue	93	35 (38)
Bone	60	10 (17)
Lung parenchyma	32	6 (19)
Liver	18	1 (6)

Drug toxicity

Overall 153 patients were assessable for 4OHA toxicity, of whom 124 (81%) had no side effects attributed to treatment. 10 (5%) patients were withdrawn from treatment because of toxicity. Side effects may be divided into those local to the administration site and systemic reactions. Of patients receiving parenteral therapy 8 developed sterile abscesses at the injection site and a further 5 experienced injection related pain. The majority (9) of these patients were in the higher dose study and included 3 of the 8 patients treated with 1 g of 4OHA weekly. 6 patients were withdrawn from treatment because of problems related to injection sites and in the majority of the others, the dose or route of administration was varied. One patient treated with oral 4OHA complained of indigestion and was withdrawn from treatment.

The majority of systemic reactions were mild and transient, and included flushing, peri-oral oedema, lethargy, drowsiness, chest pain and myalgia. Two patients developed a skin rash; one of these was withdrawn. Two patients had isolated and unrepeated anaphylactoid reactions immediately following injection after some months of treatment. One patient was discontinued because of myositis and one because of neutropenia (WBC 2.5); in both cases there was a prompt recovery on cessation of treatment.

The low incidence of side effects experienced by patients treated with 4OHA may be compared to the incidence of adverse reaction associated with aminoglutethimide treatment. Between 40 and 80% of patients receiving aminoglutethimide complain of side effects, particularly lethargy and drowsiness, nausea and skin rash [8, 17, 33].

Endocrine studies

We have studied the endocrine effects of 4OHA both in single dose studies and during continued treatment [13, 14, 16, 34]. Plasma concentrations of oestradiol, 4OHA and other hormones were measured by radioimmunoassay.

The major endocrine effect of 4OHA administration is a reduction in the plasma oestradiol concentration. The apparent failure of plasma oestrogen levels, as measured by radioimmunoassay, to fall significantly, which we reported in an early study [16], was surprising. We believe this to be the result of cross-reaction in the radioimmunoassay since we have now shown that when measured by gas chromatography – mass spectrometry oestrone levels are suppressed by a means value of 60% [14, 15].

Following a single injection of 500 mg of 4OHA, serum oestradiol fell to a nadir of 36.3 ± 3.3% (SEM) (n = 14) of the pretreatment concentration by 4 to 7 days following administration; in the majority of patients suppression was maintained for more than 14 days. A similar degree of oestradiol suppression was seen during daily administration of 500 mg of 4OHA by mouth for 7 days and following single injections of 125 mg of 4OHA but recovery of serum oestradiol concentrations occurred more rapidly. The half life of plasma 4OHA, following intramuscular injection, is approximately 8 days, compared to approximately 2½ hours following an oral dose. This suggests that there is a depot effect following intramuscular injection.

During chronic administration of 4OHA, oestradiol suppression is maintained. No difference in the degree of oestradiol suppression for responding and non responding patients has been observed and disease progression is not associated with an escape from oestradiol suppression in previously responding patients. Oestradiol levels were reduced to a mean of 37.1 ± 4.9% of baseline in 11 patients treated with the dose of 500 mg im. weekly and to 44.5 ± 7.9% of baseline in 6 patients taking the oral dose. In 13 patients treated with 250 mg im. every 2 weeks, oestradiol levels were suppressed to a mean of 40.6 ± 6.8% of the pretreatment value after one week. At the end of the second week, the levels rose to 54 ± 6.4% of the pretreatment value, which is a significant increase ($p = 0.03$, paired t-test). The increase in the oestradiol levels between day 7 and day 14 of treatment suggests that the 250 mg alternate week dose regime of 4OHA may achieve marginally suboptimal aromatase inhibition during the last few days of the 2 week cycle. The clinical relevance of this is not established.

4OHA in advanced breast cancer: conclusion

4OHA appears to be free of side effects in the majority of patients whilst retaining the clinical efficiency of AG. 4OHA has not been adequately evaluated in patients who have not been previously treated with endocrine therapy.

Despite the efficacy of 4OHA more effective selective aromatase inhibitors are needed to suppress oestradiol to a greater extent than can currently be achieved.

Recently an important new compound, pyridoglutethimide, has become available. This compound, which has been synthesised by our group, is currently undergoing phase I clinical trials.

Methotrexate – mitoxantrone cytotoxic chemotherapy

Cytotoxic chemotherapy in advanced breast cancer is administered predominantly for palliation. There is little evidence that chemotherapy is able to prolong survival [30, 35]. The majority of drugs in current use cause unpleasant side effects which are likely to contribute to the poor quality of life of patients receiving cytotoxic treatment. The most active agent in breast cancer is doxorubicin which causes alopecia, emesis, stomatitis and is cardiotoxic. Even when administered at attenuated doses as part of a combination, toxicity is substantial. The development of an effective non-doxorubicin containing regime potentially offers a substantial improvement in the quality of life of patients treated with cytotoxic therapy.

The MMM regime [22, 29] consists of a combination of the anthracenedione, mitoxantrone, the alkylating antibiotic, mitomycin C and the antimetabolite, methotrexate. The MMM regime rarely causes significant alopecia and has a low emetogenic potential. In a randomised trial it has been shown to be better tolerated than but as effective as a doxorubicin based regime (VAC: vincristine, doxorubicin, cyclophosphamide). Unfortunately MMM is myelotoxic and causes a degree of cumulative myelosuppression. In an attempt to limit the myelotoxicity of the combination whilst retaining its clinical efficacy, we have omitted mitomycin C, without compensatory modification of the dose of mitoxantrone and methotrexate. We present below a preliminary analysis of our trial of MM vs MMM in advanced breast cancer which is currently in progress.

To date 50 patients, all of whom had previously been treated with at least one endocrine treatment for advanced disease have been entered into the study. Five patients only had received prior cytotoxic chemotherapy. The population of patients treated was relatively elderly (median age 64, range 30 – 87) and had relatively poor performance scores (median Karnofsky 70, range 40 – 90). The treatment schedule is shown in table 9. Patients randomised to the MMM arm have tended to be slightly older and have poorer performance scores than those receiving MM. We have used standard staging procedures prior to entry and on completion and have used UICC criteria to assess response.

43 patients have been evaluated for response; 7 patients remain on treatment. The overall response details, and the numbers of patients responding according to disease site are shown in table 10. The overall response rate is relatively low, probably because of the poor prognosis of patients entered, but seems to be

Table 9 Treatment schedule

Methotrexate 30 mg/m^2 every 3 weeks Mitroxantrone 6 – 7 mg/m^2 every 3 weeks	vs	Methotrexate 30 mg/m^2 every 3 weeks Mitoxantrone 6 – 7 mg/m^2 every 3 weeks Mitomycin C 6 – 7 mg/m^2 every 6 weeks

6 cycles administered

Folinic acid rescue not routinely used

Dexamethasone ± Domperidone used as routine first-line antiemetic therapy

Table 10 MM vs. MMM: response

	MM	MMM
Number assessable	22	21
CR/PR	8 (36%)	6 (29%)
NC	7	6
PD	7	9

6 patients crossed from MM to MMM because of inadequate response: 1 patient had PR after cross-over

Response according to disease site

	MM	MMM
Soft tissue	5/20	4/17
Bone	4/15	4/15
Lung Parenchyma	0/3	0/6
Liver and Other Viscera	2/9	1/9

comparable in the 2 arms. 6 patients were crossed over from MM to MMM because of inadequate response to MM; one patient who had a mixed response to MM had a partial response on crossing over to MMM.

Non-haematological toxicity was similar, in our study, to the previously reported trial of MMM, with only 3 patients developing severe emesis, and one patient alopecia. 12 patients complained of minor lethargy and 3 of severe lethargy. There was one case of non-fatal cardiac toxicity. No difference was seen between the 2 arms of the study.

Table 11 MM vs. MMM: haematological toxicity

	MM	MMM
Number of patients experiencing neutropenic infection	1	8
Number of treatment related deaths	0	1
Number of patients requiring dose reduction/delay for neutropenia	3	6
Number of patients requiring dose reduction/delay for thrombocytopenia	0	1
Nadir WBC on 1st cycle		
$>3 \times 10^9$/L	13	9
2–3	2	5
1–2	2	4
<1	0	7
Nadir platlets on 1st cycle		
$\leq 100 \times 10^9$/L	2	2

MM chemotherapy appears to be associated with substantially less haematological toxicity than MMM (table 11). The number of patients with nadir leucocyte counts $< 2 \times 10^9$/1 on the first cycle, the number of patients experiencing neutropenic infection and the number of patients requiring a dose reduction or delay because of haematological toxicity were all greater in the MMM arm than in the MM arm. The one treatment related death occurred in a patient who refused to seek medical help when she became ill, presumably from sepsis after her first injection of MMM chemotherapy.

Our preliminary results suggest that MM chemotherapy is as effective at palliation of advanced breast cancer and is associated with significantly less haematological toxicity than MMM chemotherapy. Both regimes appear to offer a significant advance over anthracycline based regimes in terms of reduced toxicity. The MM regime may prove suitable for adjuvant treatment of primary breast cancer.

References

[1] Berger, U., J. L. Mansi, P. Wilson et al.: Detection of estrogen receptor in bone marrow from patients with metastatic breast cancer. J. Clin. Oncol. 5 (1987) 1179–1182.

[2] Brodie, A. M. H., W. C. Schwarzel, H. J. Brodie: Studies on the mechanism of estrogen biosynthesis in the rat ovary. J. Steroid Biochem. 7 (1976) 787–793.

[3] Brodie, A. M. H., W. C. Schwarzel, A. A. Shikh et al.: The effect of an aromatase inhibitor 4-hydroxy-4-androstene-3, 17-dione on estrogen-dependent processes in reproduction and breast cancer. Endocrinology *100* (1977) 1684–1695.

[4] Brodie, A. M. H., L.-Y. Wing, P. Goss et al.: Aromatase inhibitors and the treatment of breast cancer. J. Steroid Biochem. *24* (1986) 91 – 97.

[5] Coombes, R. C., D. P. Dearnaley, W. H. Redding et al.: Micrometastases in breast cancer. In: H. Peeters (ed.): Protides of the Biological Fluids, pp. 317 – 323. Pergamon Press, Oxford 1983.

[6] Coombes, R. C., P. E. Goss, M. Dowsett et al.: 4-Hydroxyandrostenedione in the treatment of postmenopausal patients with advanced breast cancer. Lancet *2* (1984) 1237 – 1239.

[7] Coombes, R. C., T. J. Powles, M. Abbott et al.: Physical tests for distant metastases in patients with breast cancer. J. Roy. Soc. Med. *73* (1980) 617 – 623.

[8] Coombes, R. C., T. J. Powles, D. Easton et al.: Adjuvant aminoglutethimide therapy for postmenopausal patients with primary breast cancer. Cancer Res. *47* (1986) 2496 – 2499.

[9] Cunningham, D., T. J. Powles, M. Dowsett et al.: Oral 4-hydroxyandrostenedione, a new endocrine treatment for disseminated breast cancer. Cancer Chemother. Pharmacol. *20* (1987) 253 – 255.

[10] Dearnaley, D. P., M. G. Ormerod, J. P. Sloane et al.: Detection of isolated mammary carcinoma cells in marrow of patients with primary breast cancer. J. Roy. Soc. Med. *76* (1983) 359 – 364.

[11] Dearnaley, D. P., J. P. Sloane, M. G. Ormerod et al.: Increased detection of mammary carcinoma cells in marrow smears using antisera to epithelial membrane antigen. Br. J. Cancer. *44* (1981) 85 – 90.

[12] Delsol, G., K. C. Gatter, H. Stein et al.: Human lymphoid cells express epithelial membrane antigen: implication for diagnosis of human neoplasms. Lancet *2* (1984) 1124 – 1128.

[13] Dowsett, M., P. E. Goss, T. J. Powles et al.: Use of the aromatase inhibitor 4-hydroxyandrostenedione in postmenopausal breast cancer; optimisation of therapeutic dose and route. Cancer Res. *47* (1987) 1957 – 1961.

[14] Dowsett, M., D. Cunningham, S. Evans et al.: Aromatase inhibitor 4-hydroxyandrostenedione in breast cancer: endocrinology and dose optimisation of oral and parenteral routes. In: F. Bresciani, R.-B. King, Mc' Lippman, J.-P. Raynaud (ed.): Progress in Cancer Research and Therapy, Vol. *35*: Hormones and Cancer 3, pp. 318 – 325. Raven Press, New York 1988.

[15] Dowsett, M., D. C. Cunningham, R. C. Stein et al.: Dose-related endocrine effects and pharmacokinetics of oral and intramuscular 4-hydroxyandrostenedione in postmenopausal breast cancer patients. Cancer Res. 49 (1989) 1306 – 1312.

[16] Goss, P. E., T. J. Powles, M. Dowsett et al.: Treatment of advanced postmenopausal breast cancer with an aromatase inhibitor, 4-hydroxyandrostenedione: phase II report. Cancer Res. *46* (1986) 4823 – 4826.

[17] Harris, A. L., T. J. Powles, I. E. Smith: Aminoglutethimide in the treatment of advanced postmenopausal breast cancer. Cancer Res. *42* (1982) 3405 s – 3408 s.

[18] Hayward, J. L., P. P. Carbone, J.-C. Heuson et al.: Assessment of response to therapy in advanced breast cancer. Cancer *39* (1977) 1289 – 1294.

[19] Heyderman, E., K. Steele, M. G. Ormerod: A new antigen on the epithelial membrane: its immunoperoxidase localisation in normal and neoplastic tissue. J. Clin. Pathol. *32* (1979) 35 – 39.

[20] Ingle, J. N., D. C. Tormey, H. K. Tan: The bone marrow examination in breast cancer. Cancer *41* (1978) 670–674.

[21] Jaffe, H. L.: Tumors metastatic to the skeleton. In: Tumors and tumorous conditions of the bones and joints, pp. 589–618. Lea and Febiger, Philadelphia 1968.

[22] Judson, I. R.: Mitomycin C, Mitozantrone and methotrexate (MMM) used in combination as effective, well tolerated chemotherapy of disseminated breast cancer. In: Proceedings of the 3rd United Kingdom Novantrone Symposium, pp. 73–80. Media Medica, Chichester 1988.

[23] King, W. J., G. L. Greene: Monoclonal antibodies localize estrogen receptor in the nuclei of target cells. Nature *307* (1984) 745–747.

[24] McClelland, R. A., U. Berger, L. S. Miller et al.: Immunocytochemical assay for estrogen receptor in patients with breast cancer: relationship to a biochemical assay and to outcome of therapy. J. Clin. Oncol. *4* (1986) 1171–1176.

[25] McClelland, R. A., U. Berger, P. Wilson et al.: Presurgical determination of estrogen receptor status using immunocytochemically stained fine needle aspirate smears in patients with breast cancer. Cancer Res. *47* (1987) 6118–6122.

[26] McGuire, W. L., M. DeLaGarza: Improved sensitivity in the measurement of estrogen receptor in human breast cancer. J. Clin. Endocrinol. Metab. *37* (1973) 986–989.

[27] Mansi, J. L., U. Berger, D. Easton et al.: Micrometastases in bone marrow in patients with primary breast cancer: evaluation as an early predictor of bone metastases. Br. Med. J. *47* (1987) 1093–1096.

[28] Ormerod, M. G., K. Steele, J. H. Westwood et al.: Epithelial membrane antigen: partial purification, assay and properties. Br. J. Cancer. *48* (1983) 533–541.

[29] Powles, T. J., S. E. Ashley, G. V. Forgeson et al.: Treatment of advanced breast cancer with mitomycin-C, mitoxantrone and methotrexate (3M) compared to vincristine, adriamycin and cyclophosphamide (VAC), in G. Bonadonna (ed.) Clinical Progress with Mitoxantrone pp. 1–7, Royal Society of Medicine, London, 1987.

[30] Powles, T. J., I. E. Smith, H. T. Ford et al.: Failure of chemotherapy to prolong survival in a group of patients with metastatic breast cancer. Lancet *1* (1980) 580–582.

[31] Ridell, B., K. Landys: Incidence and histopathology of metastases of mammary carcinoma in biopsies from the posterior iliac crest. Cancer *44* (1979) 1782–1788.

[32] Sloane, J. P., D. P. Dearnaley, M. G. Ormerod: Epithelial membrane antigen and lymphoid cells. Lancet *1* (1985) 109–110.

[33] Smith, I. E., A. L. Harris, M. Morgan et al.: Tamoxifen versus aminoglutethimide in advanced breast cancer: a randomised cross-over trial. Br. Med. J. *283* (1981) 1432–1434.

[34] Stein, R. C., M. Dowsett, A. Hedley et al.: Treatment of advanced breast cancer in post-menopausal women with 4-hydroxyandiostenedione. Cancer Chemother. Pharmacol. (1989, in press).

[35] Vincent, M. D., T. J. Powles, R. Skeet et al.: An analysis of possible prognostic features of long-term and short-term survivors of metastatic breast cancer. Eur. J. Cancer Clin. Oncol. *22* (1986) 1059–1065.

Prognostic factors in cancer clinical trials – some recent methodological developments

A. Neiß

Introduction

"Prognostic factors" are factors which statistically influence the effects of treatment. These factors should be accounted for in planning, evaluating, and interpreting the results of clinical trials. Depending on the objective of the trial, this may be done in various ways. The following three questions regarding prognostic factors will be examined in this paper:

- identifying prognostic factors
- accounting for prognostic factors in statistical analysis
- analyzing interactions between prognostic factors and treatment.

In all three areas new approaches have been developed and new understandings have been gained.

Identifying prognostic factors

Often many variables must be analysed to determine which influence the result of treatment. There are two ways to approach this problem: either the univariate method or the multivariate method. In the univariate method one checks each variable separately as to whether there is a correlation between the variable and the effect of treatment. In the multivariate approach a mathematical model is used which analyses all competing variables simultaneously; it describes the relationship between prognostic factors and the effects of treatment. In cancer trials, two different methods are used depending on the variable used to measure the effects of treatment: multiple logistic regression for alternative variables (e. g. yes/no questions) and COX's regression model for time variables. The analysis as to whether a certain variable can be regarded as a prognostic factor is performed by statistical tests which use so-called model parameters.

Usually the potential prognostic factors can be assessed at the beginning of the study. Sometimes, however, the investigator wants to know, for example, whether achievement of remission is a prognostic factor determining time to progression or survival time. In this case the investigator does not know in advance whether a remission will occur or not. The variable can only be assessed after treatment has begun.

This accounts for there being a bias in the results of the statistical analysis: If, for example, survival time is the object of interest and remission is defined as a certain improvement occurring within two months of commencing treatment, then all deaths occurring within these two months will be classified under the heading "no remission", i. e., this group is at a disadvantage by definition.

The expected systematic error is called "guarantee time bias", "responder versus non-responder bias" or "time until response bias". This problem was noticed for the first time in the course of an analysis of heart transplant data, which was designed to determine whether patients who had undergone transplantation were living longer than those who had not undergone transplantation [3, 6, 10]. In this case too, a certain group is systematically at a disadvantage: all patients who had died before the intended transplantation are attributed to the group of patients who had not undergone transplantation.

Statistically one can solve this problem by including the variable "remission" as a time-dependent covariable in COX's model. The variable is 0, if no remission has occurred, and becomes 1 when remission is diagnosed.

Simon and Makuch [9] proposed another approach: they used the mathematical model proposed by Mantel and Byar [6] and Aalen [1]. The state of a patient is modelled as a continuous time, non-homogeneous, Markov process. This method leads to the same results as the approach using a time-dependent covariate. Simon and Makuch also modified the procedure of Kaplan and Meier [5] for graphical presentation of data.

Using these methods the investigator does not have to regard the variable "remission" as a factor whose value is set at the beginning of treatment and can thus avoid a systematic error.

Accounting for prognostic factors

Since prognostic factors influence the result of treatment, a study comparing different therapies has to be planned and evaluated in such a way that these influences do not bias the result of treatment comparison. Usually patients are randomly allocated to the various treatment groups. A stratified randomization can also be used. The aim of randomization is to achieve comparability of treatment groups according to their prognostic factors. During evaluation, regression models can be used in order to avoid a bias. Another possibility is post-stratification.

Usually simple randomization eliminates the negative influence of prognostic factors sufficiently. This is no longer true when a time variable is used to measure treatment success (e. g. time to progression, survival time) as is in the case of most cancer clinical trials. Schumacher, Olschewski, and Schmoor [7] showed that in the course of a non-stratified comparison of treatments a systematic error may occur even when randomization has been carried out correctly. This is caused by the heterogeneity of the treatment groups due to different values of the prognostic factors for each patient. In the course of the treatment, the distribution of prognostic factors within the treatment groups will change. For example patients with unfavourable prognostic factors will die earlier, so that the proportion of patients with favorable prognosis will increase during the study. If the effects of the treatments are different, this development will proceed differently in the various treatment groups. If one considers two therapies, this means that the relative risk changes with time. Several statistical procedures, however, (e. g., the logrank test) demand that this ratio remain constant during the course of the study. According to Schumacher et al. [7] one has to expect treatment differences being underestimated when using these methods.

Consequently, the investigator should include the relevant prognostic factors in the statistical analysis either by post-stratification followed by a stratified logrank test or by handling these variables as covariates in COX's regression model.

Analyzing interactions between prognostic factors and treatment

Apart from the identification of prognostic factors and the elimination of their influence in comparisons of different treatments, analysis of the effects of these factors is also of interest. In clinical trials the question as to whether the difference between the effects of treatments depends on a prognostic factor is often examined. One then speaks of an interaction between treatment effect and prognostic factor. This question is important, for example, in determining whether a subgroup of patients which benefits of a new treatment to a larger extent than the remaining patients can be defined.

In order to detect interactions, two procedures can be used: a mathematical model (e. g., logistic regression or COX's model) or subgroup analysis.

In subgroup analysis patients are classified in subgroups according to their prognostic factors, and treatment success is compared within these subgroups of the total population. This means that the individual comparisons are usually based on populations with small sample size. Consequently, it is difficult to prove significant differences. The same applies to models: additional terms for potential interactions and, therefore, further model parameters have to be integrated, which also reduces the power of the tests of significance.

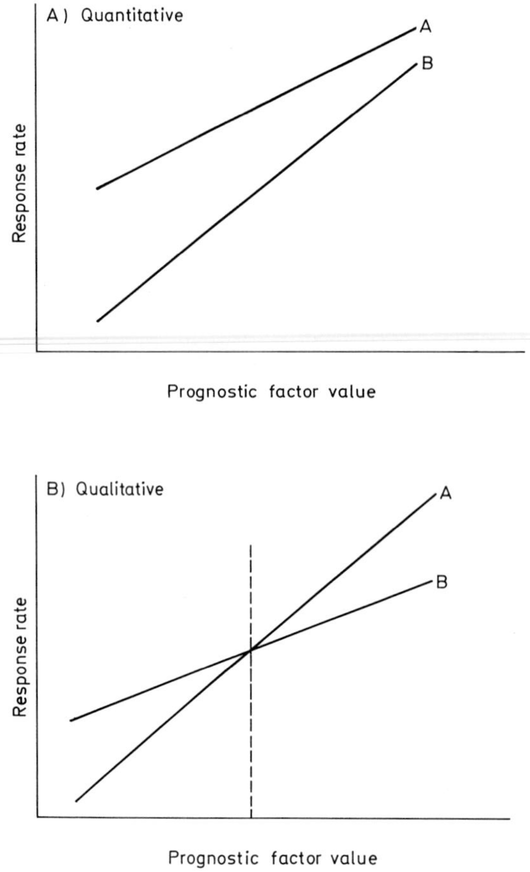

Fig. 1 Two types of treatment-covariate interactions (see text for explanation)

Two kinds of interactions can be distinguished: quantitative and qualitative interactions. In figure 1 these kinds of interactions are presented.

When the interaction is quantitative, the difference of the treatment success depends on the prognostic factor, however, one therapy (here: A) is always better than the other (here: B). When the interaction is qualitative one therapy is superior for a certain range of values of the prognostic factor (here: for small values of the prognostic factor: therapy B) and the other therapy is superior for the other range (here: for large values of the prognostic factor: therapy A).

Although in practice qualitative interactions are of greater interest than quantitative interactions, the procedures discussed so far do not distinguish between these two kinds of interactions. Qualitative interactions can be detected by models and tests of significance recently developed [2, 4, 8].

Concluding remarks

Statistical tests identify prognostic factors and interactions between prognostic factors and effects of treatment. The hypotheses to be tested can be formulated either at the beginning of the study, i. e., before the data is inspected, or afterwards, when the data is available. The first approach is called confirmative data analysis, the second one exploratory data analysis. Results of exploratory data analysis can produce false positive results. Therefore the prognostic factors or interactions identified should be carefully considered. Are there biological models, animal experiments, or other clinical trials which support these results? The results may have to be re-examined in new clinical trials.

References

[1] Aalen, O. O.: Nonparametric Inference for a Family of Counting Processes. Annals of Statistics *6* (1978) 701 – 726.

[2] Byar, D. P.: Assessing Apparent Treatment – Covariate Interactions in Randomized Clinical Trials. Statistics in Medicine *4* (1985) 255 – 263.

[3] Crowley, J., M. Hu: The Covariance Analysis of Heart Transplant Data. Journal of the American Statistical Association *72* (1977) 27 – 36.

[4] Gail, M., R. Simon: Testing for Qualitative Interactions Between Treatment Effects and Patient Subsets. Bionmetrics *41* (1985) 361 – 372.

[5] Kaplan, E. L., P. Meier: Nonparametric Estimation from Incomplete Observations. Journal of the American Statistical Association *53* (1958) 457 – 481.

[6] Mantel, N., D. P. Byar: Evaluation of Response-Time Data Involving Transient States: An Illustration Using Heart Transplant Data. Journal of the American Statistical Association *69* (1974) 81 – 86.

[7] Schumacher, M., M. Olschewski, C. Schmoor: The Impact of Heterogeneity on the Comparison of Survival Times. Statistics in Medicine *6* (1987) 773 – 784.

[8] Shuster, J., J. van Eys: Interaction Between Prognostic Factors and Treatment. Controlled Clinical Trials *4* (1983) 209 – 214.

[9] Simon, R., R. W. Makuch: A Nonparametric Graphical Representation of the Relationship Between Survival and the Occurence of an Event: Application to Responder Versus Non-Responder Bias. Statistics in Medicine *3* (1984) 35 – 44.

[10] Turnbull, B. W., B. W. Brown Jr., M. Hu: Survivorship Analysis of Heart Transplant Data. Journal of the American Statistical Association *69* (1974) 74 – 80.

Prognosis-adapted treatment strategy in metastatic breast cancer

K. Possinger, W. Wilmanns

Introduction

In patients with metastasized breast cancer curative therapy is beyond our reach at present. This fact compels us to balance the possible reduction of the tumour load induced by the cytotoxic therapy against the drug related toxicity the patient has to cope with.

The extraordinary variety of the courses of disease in patients with metastasized breast cancer has been known for many years. Therefore the claim is that the form and intensity of a systemic therapy should be adapted to the individual prognosis of the patient. The relevance of prognostic factors has been pointed out again and again in many studies [1–5]. The disease-free interval, the localisation and the number of metastatic sites, the estrogen and progesterone receptor content of the tumour cells and the performance status of the patients are considered the most important prognostic factors. Together they indicate a favourable or unfavourable course of disease [6]. Nevertheless, it is seldom that one finds prospective randomized studies in the literature where treatment modalities are based on prognostic parameters. Additionally, there is a striking lack of studies which grade the importance of the prognostic factors.

Prognosis-adapted therapeutic strategy

Therefore in our hospital we performed a study evaluating the survival time and the effect of the first polychemotherapy on the course of disease. 501 patients with histologically proven breast cancer and distant metastases not manageable otherwise (surgery/irradiation) entered the study; 475 patients are evaluable for response; median follow-up is now 6.5 years. The patients were distributed into groups with favourable and unfavourable prognostic factors. For statistical evaluation we developed a prognostic score based mainly on clinical experience. For practical reasons we decided to consider only the disease-free interval, the site

Prognostic Factors	*Points*
Site	
Skin, Soft Tissue	1
Bone, Effusion	1
Lung: nodular	
solitary	3
multiple	5
Lymphangiosis ca.	6
Liver	6
Bone Marrow	4
Receptor-Status	
positive	1
unknown	2
negative	3
Relapse-free Interval	
> 2 years	1
< = 2 years	3

Favourable Prognosis:	*< 7 Points*
Unfavourable Prognosis:	*> = 7 Points*

Med. Klinik III. GH. K. P. 318 – 88

Fig. 1 Prognostic score

of metastases and the receptor status (fig. 1). Patients with 7 or more score points were classified to the high risk group, patients with less than 7 points to the low risk group.

In patients with a favourable prognosis and positive or unknown hormonal receptor status, we started with hormonal treatment: In premenopausal patients we performed an oophorectomy and in postmenopausal patients we administered tamoxifen. Premenopausal patients relapsing from an initial hormonal treatment received tamoxifen and the postmenopausal high doses of MPA (Medroxyprogesterone acetate). Patients with negative hormonal receptor status or with tumour progression under hormonal therapy were put onto a CMF-regimen (cyclophosphamide, methotrexate, 5-fluorouracil).

In patients with unfavourable prognosis we administered a combination of vincristine, adriamycin and cyclophosphamide as first-line chemotherapy. Pre-

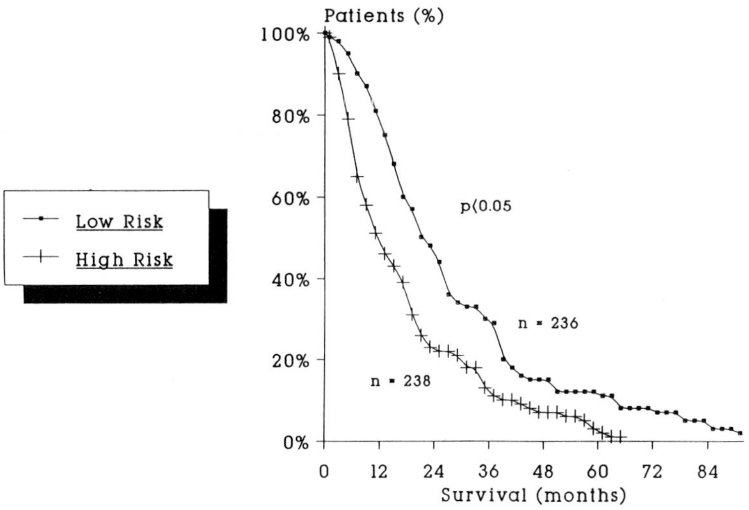

Fig. 2 Survival time calculated from the first occurrence of distant metastases

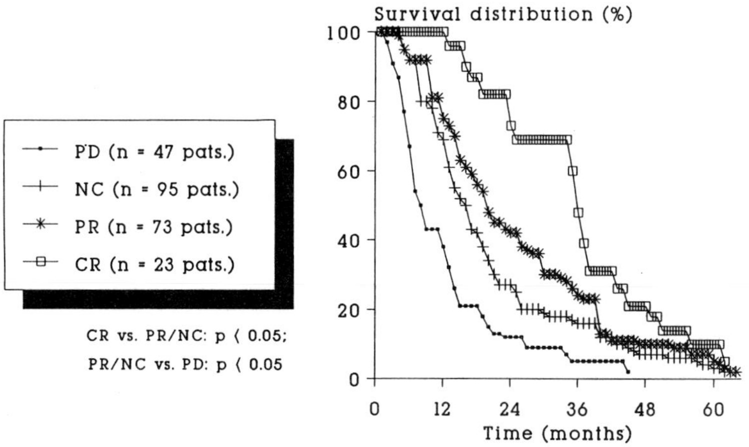

Fig. 3 Survival time of low risk patients calculated from the first occurrence of distant metastases

menopausal patients with positive or unknown hormonal receptor status were additionally oophorectomized, postmenopausal women received tamoxifen.

The usefulness of our prognostic score was shown in measuring the survival time of the two patient groups (fig. 2): Patients with favourable prognostic criteria survived a median of 22 months from the first occurence of distant metastases. Patients with unfavourable criteria only a median of 12 months. The survival times of the two groups differed significantly ($p<.05$). Looking at the relevance for survival of the response to the first combination chemotherapy, we found considerable differences between the two groups.

Patients with favourable prognostic criteria (fig. 3) had exactly the same survival time, independent of tumour progression, stable disease or even partial remission; only patients with complete remission survived longer. But the number of patients with complete remission was very low (18/237 pts.).

Analyzing these results, we had to state, that most of our patients with a favourable prognosis had been overtreated: Only in some patients did polychemotherapy improve the quality of life by reducing tumour related symptoms. All the others had to bear the marked toxicity of polychemotherapy for months without achieving a prolongation of survival time from this treatment, except the few patients with complete tumour remission.

In patients with unfavourable prognostic factors (fig. 4) the impact of the therapeutic efficacy of the initial chemotherapy on survival time was completely different: Patients with primary tumour progression survived significantly less time ($p<.05$) than patients showing stable disease or partial remission. Complete remission paralleled with the longest survival time. In contrast to the low risk group most patients with unfavourable prognostic factors apparently benefitted from chemotherapy: 191 of 238 patients achieving stable disease, partial or complete tumour remission had a significantly longer survival time than those patients with immediate tumour progression. In addition to this, in most of the patients in this group, polychemotherapy induced at least a transient stabilisation or an improvement of tumour induced symptoms.

Analysis: CNF vs. CAF

Some months ago we had access to the data of a large international prospective randomized first line polychemotherapy trial [5] comparing CAF (cyclophosphamide, adriamycin, 5-fluorouracil) versus CNF (cyclophosphamide, mitoxantrone, 5-fluorouracil). In this trial more than 300 patients were enrolled. The aim of the study was to compare the efficacy and the acute and subacute toxicity of two polychemotherapies (5-fluorouracil, adriamycin, cyclophosphamide versus 5-fluorouracil, mitoxantrone, cyclophosphamide).

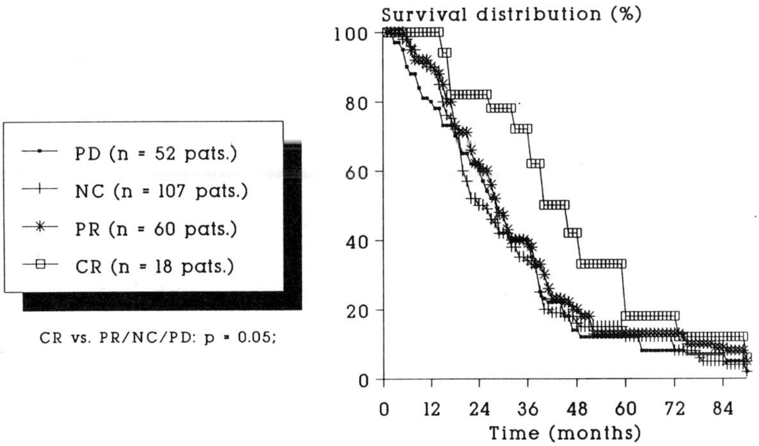

Fig. 4 Survival time of high risk patients calculated from the first occurrence of distant metastases

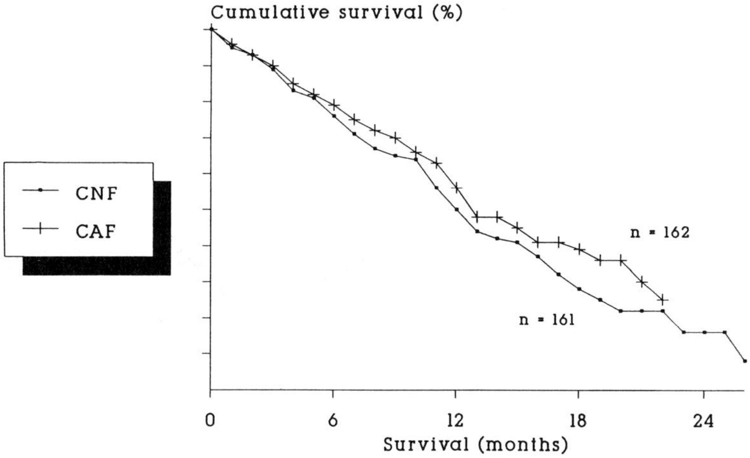

Fig. 5 Survival time calculated from the first occurrence of distant metastases (CAF vs. CNF)

Even in this study the characteristics of the patients (age, number and site of the metastases, performance status etc.) were well balanced, and even the response rates, the response duration and the survival time did not differ in both treatment arms (fig. 5). Using our prognostic score we were again able to separate two groups of patients with statistically significant survival time ($p<.05$): Patients classified into the "low risk" group survived a median of 22 months, whereas

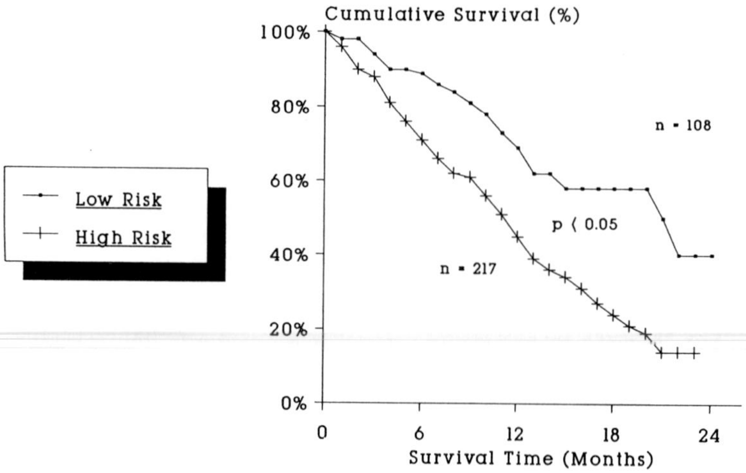

Fig. 6 Survival time calculated from the first occurrence of distant metastases (CAF vs. CNF)

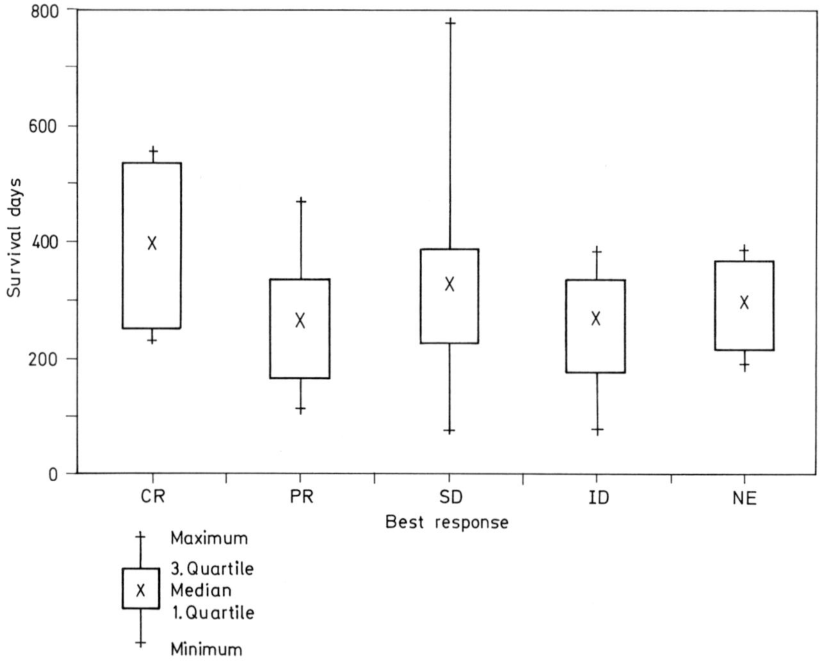

Fig. 7 Low risk patients: correlation between the best response to first chemotherapy (CAF/CNF) and survival.

CR = complete remission
PR = partial remission
SD = stable disease
ID = progressive disease
NE = not evaluable

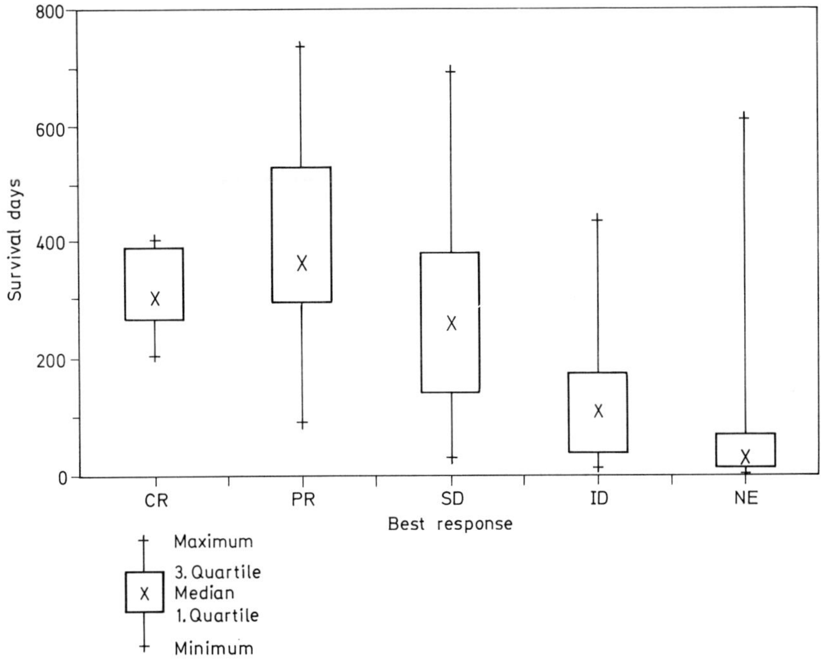

Fig. 8 High risk patients: correlation between the best response to first chemotherapy (CAF/CNF) and survival.
CR = complete remission
PR = partial remission
SD = stable disease
ID = progressive disease
NE = not evaluable

"high risk"-patients survived only a median of 13 months (fig. 6). Correlating the efficacy of first line chemotherapy with survival, we got the same results: in patients with favourable prognostic factors there was again no correlation between response to chemotherapy and survival (fig. 7).

We do not know if in these patients polychemotherapy was administered by routine or, in order to ameliorate obvious tumour induced symptoms, not manageable otherwise. And we also do not know, how many patients benefitted from this therapy by alleviating their complaints, but we have to consider that the measurable response to the chemotherapy had no measurable impact on survival. In patients classified into the "high risk"-group we found results similar to our study (fig. 8): Patients with tumour progression, in spite of chemotherapy, survived significantly less time than patients with disease stabilisation or objective remission.

Consequences for a new prognosis-adapted therapeutic strategy

To reduce the toxicity of chemotherapy we planned a multicenter trial based on a prognosis orientated, disease adapted therapeutic strategy: In patients with favourable prognostic factors and positive or unknown hormonal receptor status, to avoid the morbidisation due to oophorectomy, additive hormonal treatment is initiated: premenopausal patients receive chemical castration by gonadotropin releasing hormone analogues or antagonists, postmenopausal women are treated with tamoxifen; patients showing stabilisation or remission of tumour growth receive a second hormonal treatment at relapse; premenopausal patients then receive tamoxifen and postmenopausal women aminoglutethimide or medroxyprogesterone acetate. Patients with negative hormonal receptor status or progression under hormonal treatment receive chemotherapy at the appearance of obvious tumour symptoms.

In a randomized study we are comparing monochemotherapy with conventional polychemotherapy. This approach seems to be justified because on the one hand we could not find a significant impact on survival from polychemotherapy in this group of patients in our study and because also in the literature a prolongation of survival could be demonstrated only in "high risk" patients [7–9].

"High risk" patients will be treated with polychemotherapy; additive hormonal treatment will be used only in premenopausal patients with positive hormonal receptor status. The type of first line chemotherapy – CMF or an anthracycline containing combination – seems not to be of relevance for remission rates or survival time [10]. First line polychemotherapies induce objective remissions in 40–70% of the patients; second line treatments are effective in 15–30% of the patients independent of a poly- or monochemotherapy. Therefore we are randomizing these second line patients between mono- and polychemotherapy.

Summary

The fact that curative treatment of advanced breast cancer is still beyond our reach, stresses the claim to reduce overall toxicity of systemic treatment. This seems to be possible by a treatment strategy, adapting the form and intensity of the therapy to the prognosis and stage of the disease and using drugs exhibiting high antitumoral efficacy combined with low systemic toxicity. In 475 patients with metastasized breast cancer we initiated a prognosis oriented therapeutic strategy: To classify patients into the high and low risk group respectively, we developed a prognostic score. Using this score we were able to separate two groups of patients showing statistically different survival times. In addition to this we found in both studies that the impact of the first polychemotherapy on survival is absolutely different in patients with favourable and unfavourable prognosis: patients with favourable prognostic factors had exactly the same survival time independent of tumour progression, stable disease or even partial remission; only patients with complete remission survived longer; in contrast, patients with unfavourable prognostic factors apparently benefitted from chemotherapy: patients achieving stable disease or objective tumour remission had a significant longer survival time than those patients with immediate tumour progression; in addition to this in most of the patients in this group, chemotherapy induced a transient stabilisation or improvement of tumour induced symptoms. Therefore, we conclude that chemotherapy of advanced breast cancer is necessary, but, in order to reduce overall toxicity, it must be planned and administered according to the individual prognostic picture.

References

[1] Alanko, A., E. Heinonen, Th. Scheinin et al.: Significance of estrogen and progesterone receptors, disease-free interval, and site of first metastasis on survival of breast cancer patients. Cancer *56* (1985) 1696 – 1700.

[2] Decker, D. A., D. L. Ahmann, H. F. Bisel et al.: Complete responders to chemotherapy in metastatic breast cancer. Characterization and analysis. JAMA *242* (1979) 2075 – 2079.

[3] Fey, M. F., K. W. Brunner, R. W. Sonntag: Prognostic factors in metastatic breast cancer. Cancer Clin. Trials *4* (1981) 237 – 247.

[4] Hortobagyi, G. N., T. L. Smith, S. S. Legha et al.: Multivariate analysis of prognostic factors in metastatic breast cancer. J. Clin. Oncol. *1* (1983) 776 – 786.

[5] Powles, T. J., I. E. Smith, H. T. Ford et al.: Failure of chemotherapy to prolong survival in a group of patients with metastatic breast cancer. Lancet *1* (1980) 580 – 582.

[6] Possinger, K.: Mammakarzinom. In: D. Huhn (ed.): Zytostatikatherapie maligner Erkrankungen, pp. 196 – 224. Gustav Fischer Verlag, Stuttgart 1986.

[7] Chlebowski, R. T., L. E. Irwin, R. P. Pugh et al.: Survival of patients with metastatic breast cancer treated with either combination or sequential chemotherapy. A Western Cancer Study Group Project. Cancer Res. *39* (1979) 4503 – 4506.

[8] Rozencweig, M., M. J. Staquet, D. D. VonHoff et al.: Prognostic factors for the response to chemotherapy in advanced breast cancer. Cancer Clin. Trials *2* (1979) 165 – 170.

[9] Hoogstraten, B., S. L. George, B. Samal et al.: Combination chemotherapy and adriamycin in patients with advanced breast cancer. A Southwest Oncology Group Study, Cancer *38* (1976) 13 – 20.

[10] Nash, C. H., S. E. Jones, T. E. Moon et al.: Prediction of outcome in metastatic breast cancer treated with Adriamycin combination chemotherapy. Cancer *46* (1980) 2380 – 2388.

Prognostic and predictive factors in breast cancer

M. Kaufmann

The main objective of the treatment of metastatic breast cancer is palliation. Because of the heterogeneous course of this chronic disease we need factors which help us to individualize and optimize therapy. There is a relationship between prognostic variables and treatment effects. In general, prognosis depends on patient, tumor, and treatment characteristics. For primary as well as for metastatic breast cancer some prognostic factors are well known and included in the therapeutic strategy [1, 6–10].

In table 1 clinically established and newly proposed prognostic factors are summarized for primary breast cancer treatment. For standard care the number of involved axillary lymph nodes in addition to steroid hormone receptors are the most important prognostic factors [3, 5].

Nuclear and histological grading, even today, are methods influenced by subjective results. The estimation of the proliferative rate (thymidine labelling index (TLI), S-phase fraction) or data on ploidy status became more relevant. Information on bone marrow infiltration, epithelial growth factor receptors (EGF-R), oncogene-amplifications or on multiple-drug resistance of breast cancer cells have become new prognostic tools.

Table 1 Prognostic factors for primary breast cancer treatment

Prognostic factor	Prognosis	
	good	poor
No. of involved nodes	0	1–3 4–9 10+
steroid hormone receptors	positive	negative
nuclear/histological grade	low/well diff.	high/poor diff.
proliferative rate (TLI, S-phase)	low	high
ploidy	diploid	aneuploid
EGF-R	negative	positive
oncogene-amplification	no	yes
multiple-drug resistance	no	yes

Table 2 Prognostic factors for metastatic breast cancer treatment

Prognostic factor	Prognosis good	poor
Patient:		
– performance status (e. g. Karnofsky-Index, WHO grade)	good	poor
– age/menopausal status	>50/postm. (>5 years)	<50/praem.
– symptoms	asymptomatic	symptomatic
– blood chemistry/tumor markers (e. g. CEA, CA 15-3, ESR)	normal	abnormal
Tumor:		
– steroid receptors	positive	negative
– No. of metastases (tumor mass)	single	multiple
– site of metastases (dominant)	s. table 3	
– disease-free interval	>2 years	<2 years
Treatment:		
– pretreatment (adjuvant/palliative)	no	yes
– prior response	yes	no

All these prognosticators for primary cancer may also play an important role in the metastatic situation.

Table 2 outlines prognostic and predictive factors in metastatic breast cancer. The most important factors related to the patient are the performance status, disease symptoms and blood chemistry abnormalities. Steroid hormone receptors are also of prognostic value being primarily relevant for the prediction of endocrine treatment response (response rates [%] for ER + PR +: ≈ 70, ER −, PR +: ≈ 40, ER + PR −: ≈ 25; ER − PR −: ≈ 10).

Further directly tumor related prognosticators are the number and sites of metastases. Disease-free interval can be an independent prognostic factor or even influenced by treatment, e. g. adjuvant systemic or radiological treatment.

Information on prior response is more or less relevant for further response in endocrine therapy manipulations. Sites of metastases are known to be determinants for the level of risk and therefore prognosis (table 3).

Poor prognosis and survival are related to visceral metastases, e. g. to the lung, liver or brain.

The prognostic factors of locally advanced or loco-regional recurrent breast cancer are listed in table 4. Histologically clear surgical resection margins are of

Table 3 Different risk categories in metastatic breast cancer for various sites of metastases

Prognosis good	Prognosis poor
loco-regional only	soft tissue
bone only	lung (multiple, lymphatic)
ipsilat. pleura effusions	liver
nodular lung	ovary
	brain
	bone marrow

Table 4 Prognostic factors of locally advanced or loco-regional recurrent breast cancer in addition to prognosticators for the primary situation

	Prognosis	
	good	poor
tumor size/area	small (<2.5 cm)	large (>2.5 cm)
inflammatory	no	yes
surgical resection margins	negative	positive
neo-adjuvant chemo- or endocrine therapy response	yes	no
previous radiotherapy	no	yes

primary importance. Neoadjuvant systemic treatment results are of predictive value for in "vivo" chemosensitivity testing.

Information on prognostic factors can undergo spontaneous or even therapy induced changes. The proliferative rate of the tumor may change during therapy or steroid hormone receptors can vary when determined before and then after cytotoxic or endocrine treatment [2].

Prognostic and predictive factors are relevant for breast cancer management. For metastatic breast cancer treatment, a selection of effective therapies is necessary to avoid toxicity (morbidity) from ineffective toxic treatment.

In addition, in vitro or in vivo chemosensitivity assays for a drug tailored chemotherapy have to be developed [4].

Prognostic and predictive factors should be prospectively taken into account in future clinical studies.

References

[1] Cannellos, G. P.: Treatment of metastases. Selection of therapy. Prognostic factors in metastatic disease. In: J. R. Harris, S. Hellman, I. C. Henderson et al. (eds.): Breast diseases, pp. 385 – 391. Lippincott Comp., Philadelphia 1987.

[2] Jonat, W.: Steroid receptors status after treatment. In: A. Pellegrini, G. Robustelli Della Cuna, F. Pannutti, P. Pouillart, W. Jonat (eds.): Role of medroxyprogesterone in endocrine-related tumors (Vol. 3), pp. 115 – 122, Raven Press, New York 1984.

[3] Kaufmann, M.: Biochemische prognostische Faktoren beim Mammakarzinom. In: F. Kubli, G. A. Nagel, U. Kadach, M. Kaufmann (eds.): Neue Wege in der Brustkrebsbehandlung, pp. 46 – 61. Aktuelle Onkologie *8*, Zuckschwerdt, München – Bern – Wien 1984.

[4] Kaufmann, M.: Biochemical short-term predictive assay: Results of correlative trials in comparison to other assays. In: V. Hofmann, M. E. Berens, G. Martz (eds.): Predictive Drug Testing on Human Tumor Cells, pp. 151 – 160. Springer, Berlin – Heidelberg – New York 1984.

[5] Kaufmann, M., W. Jonat, H. Maass et al.: Adjuvante Therapie des operablen Mammakarzinoms. Gynäkol. Prax. *12* (1988) 523 – 530.

[6] Possinger, K., H. J. Sauer, W. Wilmanns: Chemotherapie metastasierter Mammakarzinome. Dtsch. Med. Wschr. *113* (1988) 224 – 231.

[7] Schreml, W.: 10 Jahre Therapie des Mammakarzinoms. Onkologie *9* (suppl. 2) (1986) 49 – 56.

[8] Stewart, J. F., R. D. Rubens: General prognostic factors. In: G. Bonadonna (ed.): Breast Cancer: Diagnosis and Management, pp. 141 – 167. J. Wiley a. Sons, Chichester 1984.

[9] Valagussa, P., C. Brambilla, G. Bonadonna: Advanced breast cancer: Are the traditional stratification parameters still of value when patients are treated with combination chemotherapy? Eur. J. Cancer *15* (1979) 565 – 571.

[10] Wander, H. E., G. A. Nagel (eds.): Mammakarzinome, pp. 52 – 74. Prognosefaktoren des Mammakarzinoms im metastasierendem Stadium. Zuckschwerdt, München – Bern – Wien, 4. Aufl., 1986.

Evaluation criteria of palliative treatments in clinical trials of metastatic breast cancer

K. W. Brunner

Remission rate and remission duration are adequate criteria for measuring antitumor activity in phase I/II clinical trials of a new drug or a new modality of treatment. The same is true for rate of complete remission and duration of disease-free survival for treatments which aim at cure and long term survival. Short term side effects and quality of life considerations are of secondary importance for potentially curative therapies.

For palliative treatments, especially in diseases such as metastatic breast cancer, which are very heterogeneous in their course and their symptomatology, remission rate and remission duration are very inadequate criteria for evaluation and comparison, for the following reasons:

1) Remission rate does not measure the real benefit of a palliative treatment in terms of quality of life. This is mainly determined by the relief of disease symptoms and its duration and by the side effects of the treatment. Tumor regression by itself may or may not be associated with better quality of life and therefore is insufficient to define a "good" palliative treatment.
2) This is especially true, when an increase in remission rate does not correlate with an increase in survival, as has been demonstrated in most of the clinical trials for metastatic breast cancer [4].
3) A higher remission rate is often achieved with a more intensive treatment and is therefore often associated with more toxic side effects. This has a negative effect on quality of life and may annul the positive effects of the treatment.
4) In comparative clinical trials the treatment arm with the higher remission rate is not necessarily better treatment for the majority of the patients. The treatment with the higher remission rate may benefit only a minority of the patients at the expense of other patients, which may not need the more intensive and more toxic treatment and attain similar tumor control and palliation with a less toxic therapy.
5) In diseases with a long chronic course, as it is often the case in metastatic breast cancer, an intensive initial treatment with a high remission rate may compromise the effectiveness of later therapies. This may even have unfavourable effects on survival, as it has been demonstrated in some clinical trials [3].

6) Remission duration measures time of tumor control only for remitters and depends on the definition of remission with all its deficiencies [5]. A better time parameter for the effectiveness of treatment for all treated patients is time to progression or time without progression [2].

The assessment of the true absolute or comparative value of a palliative treatment cannot be based on a global indicator of average tumor shrinkage without considering extent of symptomatic relief, toxic side effects and time of tumor control of all treated patients. An adequate assessment of a palliative treatment therefore should include these three basic elements and express them in a single treatment benefit-index.

A similar concept has recently been proposed by Gelber and Goldhirsch for adjuvant chemotherapy trials of breast cancer [3]. In this concept the authors modify crude survival time by the time spent without symptoms of disease and toxicity (TWIST). Fixed time deductions are made in an uniform way for subjective toxicity of treatment, for local recurrence (3 months) and for metastatic disease (originally 100% of all further survival after occurrence of metastatic disease). This modified survival time is used as a parameter of the real benefit for the group of patients who receive adjuvant treatment compared with the untreated control group. The somewhat schematic procedure is not suited for the comparative evaluation of palliative treatments. First, the appropriate time in the assessment of palliative treatment is not survival, but the time during which tumor growth can be controlled by a certain treatment, i. e. time to progression (TTP). Furthermore, for palliative therapies it is difficult to transform symptomatic relief and toxic side effects into time elements and add or subtract them from TTP.

Instead of that, we propose a treatment index, which is based on a scoring system for each of the three basic elements: time to progression, relief of symptoms and toxic side effects. For each month without tumor progression a certain number of points is allocated. From the total sum of these points, which expresses time to progression, points for symptomatic relief (or improvement in quality of life as judged by self evaluation of the patient) which the patient experiences in each month of treatment, are added. On the other hand, toxic side effects are scored for each month of therapy and subtracted from the sum of the other points. The final index arrived at for each patient then more realistically expresses the real benefit which a patient derives from a certain treatment. For a whole group of patients on a certain treatment arm in a randomized study a mean index can be calculated and compared with the mean index of the other treatment arm.

For the construction of the treatment index, we propose a scoring system, which is summarized in table 1.

For each month without tumor progression 4 points are allocated. For each month of treatment, disease symptoms are scored from 0 – 4, as it is done on

Table 1 Proposed method for evaluation of palliative chemotherapy

	Score
1. *Time to progression* (TTP) for each month from start of therapy	4 points per month
2. *Change in score of disease symptoms* (average of performance status, pain, fatigue etc. evaluated from 0 – 4) Improvement or deterioration compared with status at start of therapy, recorded for each month of TTP	± 0 – 4 points per month
3. *Toxicity from treatment* (average of all subjective side effects, such as nausea, vomiting, stomatitis, diarrhoe, loss of appetite, treatment related infection etc. evaluated from 0 – 4) Toxicity score for each months of TTP	– 0 – 4 points per month
Months without tumor progression × 4 points *plus* months with subjective improvement × points *minus* months with subjective deterioration × points *minus* months × points from toxicity	Total score per patient

most of the flow sheets presently used for documentation of performance status, pain, fatigue etc. An average score of the subjective disease status can be calculated for each month of treatment and compared with the initial status at the start of treatment. For each month, where the disease status is better than at the beginning, a corresponding number of positive points is allocated. If disease status worsens during treatment compared with the initial status, the negative points are substracted. Alternatively or complementary, the subjective benefit from the treatment can also be assessed by the patient himself in a linear self assessment analogue form, using the same scoring from 0 – 4.

In a similar way toxic side effects are scored from 0 – 4, as it is usually done. An average score of all subjective side effects such as nausea, vomiting, stomatitis, diarrhoe, loss of appetite, treatment-related infection etc. is given for each month of treatment and the total sum of toxic points is deducted from the overall score.

Table 2 shows, how the treatment score is recorded for a patient, who showed no tumor progression for 4½ months under treatment and who experienced considerable symptomatic relief with moderate toxic effects of the treatment.

Table 3 demonstrates two examples of a treatment index: one with a treatment result which can be judged as positive and one with a result of no real treatment benefit, even if the patient may have demonstrated a partial remission during treatment.

Table 2 Example for recording the treatment score

Date	Date (1st month)	Date (2nd month)	Date (3rd month)	Date (4th month)	Date (5th month)	TTP ± TWIST
TTP	4	4	4	4	2	18 points
Change of disease related symptoms (compared with start of therapy)	3 to 1 = + 2	1 to 0 = + 3	0 = + 3	0 to 1 = + 2	1 to 1 = + 2	+ 12 points
Symptoms from toxicity	− 1	0	− 1	− 1	− 2	− 5 points
Total score	5	7	6	5	2	25 points

Table 3 Examples of treatment indices

		Points
1) Time to progression: 8 ½ months		34
Monthly average relief of symptoms: 1 ½ points		+ 12.75
Monthly average toxicity from treatment: 2 points		− 17
	Total score	29.75
2) Time to progression: 4 months		16
No relief from symptoms 1 point deterioration for 2 months		− 2
Average toxicity during the 4 months: 2		− 8
	Total score	6

Table 4 Interpretation of treatment scores

Deterioration from treatment:	<0 points
No treatment benefit:	0 – 12 points
Moderate treatment benefit:	13 – 24 points
Good treatment benefit:	25 – 48 points
Excellent treatment benefit:	>48 points

Table 4 tentatively describes which treatment index scores can be correlated with a detrimental effect of a treatment, with a lack of real treatment benefit, or with a moderate, good or excellent palliative treatment outcome. The cut-off point for beneficial effects in this system is 12 points, which corresponds to a progression-free period of 3 months in an asymptomatic patient, who experiences no side effects from treatment.

From the cited examples it can be concluded that the proposed method for the assessment of palliative treatments is not only more realistic but also discriminates much better between palliation achieved in different treatment arms of a comparative clinical trial. The discriminative property of the method may also allow for better subgroup analysis of palliative therapies. This is very important in heterogeneous neoplastic diseases such as metastatic breast cancer, where only certain subgroups of patients may benefit from a given treatment [3].

Another advantage of the new method is its independence of the definition of tumor remission. This definition has its limitations and fallacies, as has often been demonstrated [5].

For the construction of a treatment index, no new or additional data are needed. All necessary data (except patient self evaluation) are usually recorded on chemotherapy flow sheets, but are rarely used in the overall evaluation of a treatment program. Our first experiences in using this method of therapy assessment indicate that it is simple and allows for a more realistic and quality of life-oriented comparison of different treatment options than remission rate and remission duration.

References

[1] Brunner, K. W.: Problematik randomisierter Studien zur Definition optimaler Therapien beim metastasierenden Mammakarzinom. In: G. A. Nagel (ed.): Mammakarzinome, pp. 71 – 83. Springer-Verlag, Berlin – Heidelberg – New York 1986.

[2] Carter, S. K.: The role of clinical trials. In: U. Veronesi, G. Bonadonna (eds.): Clinical Trials in Cancer Medicine, pp. 1 – 24. Academic Press 1986.

[3] Gelber, R. D., A. Goldhirsch for the Ludwig Breast Cancer Study Group: A new endpoint for the assessment of adjuvant therapy in postmenopausal woman with operable breast cancer. J. Clin. Oncol. *4* (1986) 1772 – 1779.

[4] Henderson, I. C., D. F. Hayes, S. Come et al.: New agents and new medical treatments for advanced breast cancer. Sem. in Oncol. *14* (1987) 34 – 64.

[5] Mouridsen, H. T.: Value and limitation of current criteria for assessing response. In: F. Cavalli (ed.): Endocrine Treatment of Breast Cancer II. Current Developments and New Methodologies. European School of Oncology Monograph Series, Springer Verlag, Berlin – Heidelberg – New York 1987.

Systemic medical treatment before surgery in patients with operable breast cancer

I. E. Smith

Adjuvant chemotherapy and endocrine therapy are conventionally given after surgery for early breast carcinoma. However this approach has several important disadvantages. First, there is no way of knowing whether micrometastases for the individual patient are sensitive or not to the treatment given. Second, it has been postulated that growth rates for micrometastatic disease might be more rapid than for overt clinical metastases, and that even a short delay before starting chemotherapy could result in a significant increase in total tumour cell burden. Finally, it is possible that growth factors associated with surgical wound healing might stimulate rapid growth of micrometastatic disease.

For these reasons, it has been argued that adjuvant treatment should be given before rather than after surgery (so-called "neo-adjuvant" therapy). In some neo-adjuvant studies, surgery is given immediately after chemotherapy; however, this approach rules out the possibility of using the primary as a human tumour model for predicting response to therapy. More recently, several groups including ourselves have studied the feasibility of more prolonged medical therapy prior to surgery. In addition to the advantages described above, this offers the additional possibility of drug-induced tumour regression resulting in subsequent less radical surgery.

So far we have treated 57 patients with a median age of 54 years (range 29 – 84 years). Twenty-four were premenopausal, one perimenopausal (less than 3 years since LMP) and 33 postmenopausal. All had surgically operable breast cancer: patients with inflammatory carcinoma or with fixed axillary or palpable supraclavicular nodes were excluded. Fourteen had T4 tumours, 21 T3 tumours, 20 T2 tumours and 2 T1 tumours (these last patients were included on the basis that they refused any form of surgical treatment). Forty patients had clinical N1 and 10 clinical N2 axillary nodes. Diagnosis was established by histological needle biopsy and/or cytological aspirate. Patients were staged by clinical measurement and mammography. Wherever possible all investigations were repeated 2 months after starting treatment and subsequently at 6 month intervals.

Fifteen patients were treated with combination chemotherapy (using a combination of cyclophosphamide 100 mg po Days 1 – 14, methotrexate 30 mg/m^2 iv

Day 1 & 8, and 5FU 600 mg/m^2 iv Days 1 & 8, or mitomycin-C 8 mg/m^2 iv q 6 weekly, mitozantrone 8 mg/m^2 iv q 3 weekly and methotrexate 30 mg/m^2 iv q 3 weekly). One (7%) achieved complete remission and 8 (53%) partial response, giving an overall response rate of 60%. No patients showed progressive disease while on chemotherapy. Forty-two patients were treated with tamoxifen. None achieved a complete response, and 20 (47%) achieved a partial response. Only 2 patients (5%) showed progressive disease on tamoxifen.

Subsequent local treatment was individualised depending on degreee of tumour response and patients' preferences. However, 36 patients (60%) have so far avoided the need for mastectomy. With a median follow-up time of 19 months only 7 patients (12%) have developed metastatic disease and the predicted 3 year disease-free survival is 86%.

We found accurate clinical measurement of response difficult, with a >25% inter-observer error occurring in 22% of patients. Likewise, mammographic response as defined by standard UICC criteria of >50% reduction in the product of diameters was frequently difficult. More subtle mammographic changes were frequently seen, e. g. in terms of number and intensity of microcalcifications, or degree of spiculation. It may be that new criteria for defining response mammographically are required here and we are currently investigating this. We were disappointed that no histological or cytological changes after treatment could be identified which might have predicted response to treatment.

These results indicate that operable primary breast carcinoma responds to medical treatment at least as well as locally advanced or metastatic disease. Others have reported similar findings. For example, Forrest et al. [1] reported 36 patients with >4 cm operable breast carcinomas given initial medical treatment. 12/13 (92%) responded to chemotherapy with 5 (38%) complete responders. 11/23 patients (48%) responded to endocrine therapy. In contrast to our own experience, these workers reported clinical measurement as being "very precise" and mammography correlation was "seen in all cases". Mathe et al. [3] reported a 77% overall response rate to various forms of combination chemotherapy in 25 operable patients including 8% complete remissions with negative histology, and 25% complete remissions where histology showed residual micrometastatic disease. Twenty-one (84%) of these patients underwent subsequent mastectomy. Jacquillat et al. [2] reported 205 patients with primary tumours ranging from <3 cm to advanced inflammatory carcinoma. 68% responded to chemotherapy with or without tamoxifen. Subsequent radiotherapy including irridium implants achieved 100% complete remissions. For 114 patients whose original primary measured <7 cm, a predicted 96% 5 year survival was reported. Finally, in an important randomised trial Mauriac et al. [4] compared mastectomy followed by adjuvant chemotherapy with initial chemotherapy and then adapted surgery. All patients had >3 cm primary tumours. In patients treated with chemotherapy initially, 36% achieved a complete remission and 18% a partial response giving an overall response rate of 54%. 56% of these patients subsequently had conservative surgery. No survival data are so far available from this trial.

There are important problems inherent in this approach. First, an incisional (e. g. needle) biopsy gives limited information on grade, and no information on pathological tumour size or axillary node status. Hopefully it may soon be possible to identify high risk patients justifying systemic chemotherapy on the basis of immunohistochemical staining techniques rather than axillary node status. Second, in our experience measurement of response at an early stage is difficult using clinical and mammographic techniques. Disappointingly, early histological and/or cytological changes indicating response have not been seen. We are currently investigating whether ultrasound measurements of alterations in blood flow might be helpful here. Third, patients with T3 axillary node negative tumours do very well treated conventionally with mastectomy alone, with a 75% 10 year survival [5]. It is important to be sure that such patients' prognosis is not jeopardised by this newer approach. Finally, survival benefit if any could only be confirmed by a large randomised trial, given the heterogeneous nature of "operable" breast cancer.

Despite these problems early results with medical treatment prior to surgery are encouraging in terms of response, survival and the ability to reduce the need for mastectomy. Furthermore, serial biopsies and/or aspirates of the primary tumour during therapy would offer the opportunity for biological studies investigating the nature of primary tumour response to chemotherapy and/or endocrine therapy.

References

[1] Forrest, A. P. M., P. A. Levack, U. Chetty et al.: A human tumour model. Lancet *II* (1986) 840.

[2] Jacquillat, C.: Pre-operative chemotherapy and radiotherapy in breast cancer. Abstract F, 4.8, 4th EORTC Breast Cancer Conference Proceedings, 1987.

[3] Mathe, G. et al.: Surgical and histological evaluation of response to primary combination chemotherapy in operable non-inflammatory breast cancer. Abstract F, 4.5, 4th EORTC Breast Cancer Conference Proceedings, 1987.

[4] Mauriac, L.: Randomised trial comparing mastectomy ± adjuvant chemotherapy versus first-line chemotherapy followed by adapted local regional treatment for operable breast cancer. Abstract F, 4.6, 4th EORTC Breast Cancer Conference Proceedings, 1987.

[5] Valagussa, P., G. Bonadonna, U. Veronesi: Patterns of relapse and survival following radical mastectomy. Cancer *41* (1978) 1170.

Consensus statement

1. Goals of therapy

Different members of the group would place a different emphasis on the importance of different possible endpoints (time to treatment failure, response rate, quality of life) in the treatment of metastatic breast cancer.

The endpoints for physicians in practice should be the attempt to achieve maximal palliation of the symptoms with minimal toxicity for a time as long as possible (time to progression).

The endpoint of which we think is the best objective measure of efficacy, and which is therefore of special importance for clinical trials, is time to progression.

2. Endocrine therapy

Most patients should start with endocrine therapy as their first mode of treatment when there are metastases. This is especially true for some patients such as those who are ER + or PR +. However, there are other criteria that are important as well, including factors such as the disease-free interval, sites and the number of metastases. Occasionally there also could be achieved a response in ER − patients.

A group of patients who should not receive initial endocrine therapy are those with life threatening (i. e. aggressive visceral) disease.

If it is possible, patients should have repeated measurements of receptors on metastases.

Among postmenopausal women either tamoxifen or oophorectomy (ovarian ablation) will be the (initial) approach of choice. Ovarectomy, however, remains the classical treatment. Current data from randomised trials suggest that tamoxifen and oophorectomy are equally efficacious among premenopausal women. This is an area where additional research seems indicated.

An area that also deserves further observation is the exploration of the value of GnRH agonists.

For premenopausal patients that have measurably responded to tamoxifen, the secondary therapy is ovarian ablation. Among the premenopausal women the tertiary and fourth treatment should be aminoglutethimide or progestins.

The first endocrine therapy of choice in postmenopausal women is tamoxifen.

For secondary therapies among postmenopausal women either progestins or aminoglutethimide are recommended. But the optimal sequence of these two ways is not yet exactly known and should be explored further.

Aminoglutethimide is reasonable for pre-menopausal women who have had an oophorectomy. (Of course, they might be defined as post-menopausal at that point.)

In general patients should be given a second or repeated courses of hormonal therapy on the basis of a response to the preceding therapy. However, there may be exceptions to this rule, especially in the use of ovarian ablation for pre-menopausal women after a treatment with tamoxifen. In that case the use of a second endocrine therapy might be justified in a non-responder if the patients' tumor characteristics are highly suggesting that a patient will benefit from an endocrine therapy.

Although there are individual studies which suggest for one hormonal therapy an advantage over another in individual patient settings, we are not convinced that these data are compelling enough to change our recommendations regarding the sequence in which endocrine therapy should be used.

There is no hard evidence for a dose response relationship for the use of any endocrine therapy. We see no advantage for higher than usual doses of any form of endocrine therapy.

Recommended dosages:
Tamoxifen: 20 – 30 mg/die
Aminoglutethimide: 500 mg/die
Medroxyprogesterone acetate: 300 – 500 mg/die.

The recommended dose for aminoglutethimide is 500 mg/day. Eventually it should be used in combination with hydrocortisone replacement, until newer forms of aromatase inhibitors that do not require hydrocortisone replacement are available.

At the present time there is no evidence that i. m. preparations of progestins are preferable to the oral formulations.

Despite still ongoing studies evaluating higher doses of progestins, the available data provide no justification for those alterations outside clinical trials. A minority (Bastert, Possinger, Schulz, Wilmanns) voted in favour of a high-dose progestin-therapy (1000 mg/day) even outside clinical trials.

However, for hormonal manipulations in the future plasma-level adjusted dosages may result in an improvement in therapy results.

Concerning the optimal duration of endocrine treatment, the standard practice in most parts of the world is to continue endocrine treatment till progression. Until now there are not enough data to justify the termination of the endocrine treatment at an earlier time, but this deserves additional investigation.

At the present time there is no evidence for combining endocrine therapies in routine practice. The addition of prednisone to either tamoxifen or oophorectomy deserves additional study.

At present there is no role for combining chemotherapy and endocrine therapy as a routine in the clinical practice of oncology for breast cancer patients.

Sequencing endocrine therapy and chemotherapy is an area that deserves further study.

Alternating endocrine therapies, too, are areas for further challenging investigations.

3. Chemotherapy

In general, a failure to respond to endocrine therapy in a symptomatic patient is the major criteria for the use of chemotherapy. Immediate chemotherapy may be indicated in some instances, especially in rapidly developing (i. e. ER – or aggressive visceral disease).

It is possible that there are subgroups of patients that uniquely benefit from the use of chemotherapy, with prolongation of survival as a result of the treatment with chemotherapy, but we cannot at present reliably identify these subgroups. Concerning prolongation of life, for example the subgroup may include those with life-threatening disease and especially those with extensive liver metastases or aggressive visceral disease.

The possibility also exists that some subgroups of patients may actually be harmed by the use of early aggressive chemotherapy. One subgroup represents for example especially older women with more indolent forms of disease.

Optimal first line chemotherapy in symptomatic patients will be either a single agent or a combination of drugs including cyclophosphamide, methotrexate, 5-fluorouracil, doxorubicin, mitoxantrone and mitomycin C. Vincristin is not indicated in the treatment of metastatic breast cancer. It is not established that any single combination is superior to other in palliating the symptoms of metastatic breast cancer for all patients. Furthermore it is not established that a combination of drugs is always superior to a single agent. In general combination regimes containing doxorubicin have been shown to have an overall higher response rate and/or a longer time to progression compared to regimens without doxorubicin, especially for liver and other visceral manifestations. As a result some physicians would preferentially use doxorubicin containing regimens in patients with aggressive visceral disease because of the higher probability of response.

In search for new and potentially more active drugs for the treatment of metastatic breast cancer, these substances should be ideally tested in patients with little or no prior chemotherapy, because of the demonstration of lack of activity when the same agents are used in patients with heavy previous treatment. This might ideally be done in a setting where the patient has progressive disease but relatively limited symptomatology.

There are few data regarding the treatment of patients refractory to first and second line chemotherapy programs. The third line chemotherapy is active only in a minority of patients, and if it is to be used, then it is particularly important to make sure that side effects do not overweigh potential benefits.

At the present time the optimal dose schedule for most chemotherapy combinations is not well established. Recent evidence suggests that the conventional use of p. o. cyclophosphamide with i. v. methotrexate plus 5-fluorouracil is superior to intravenous programs. This is not yet confirmed and we need to be concerned about this issue. Therefore we suggest that chemotherapy regimes should be used in their originally published forms until data from controlled clinical trials suggest that another dose-rate or dose-schedule is preferable.

The optimal duration of chemotherapy is not yet known. We recommend that patients will be treated at least to palliation of symptoms assuming that this starts to occur within the first three cycles of therapy. Chemotherapy should not be continued indefinitely. The precise optimal time between these two extremes at which chemotherapy should be discontinued is not well-known. It may be in the range of 6 to 12 months.

The importance of dose for the use of chemotherapy is also not yet known. At the present time it is our recommendation that the dosis from published studies should not be reduced for trivial reasons. At the same time we feel that it is not well established that there is any advantage for increasing dosages beyond those in published standard literature outside clinical trials.

4. Locally advanced breast cancer

Medical therapy is an acceptable initial treatment for patients with inoperable locally advanced breast cancer. The therapy used should be based on the same principles as those employed for treating metastatic disease. The use of medical therapy as initial treatment in patients with operable breast cancer remains a subject of research.

5. Prior adjuvant therapy

If the patient had prior adjuvant therapy of any type – endocrine or chemotherapy – and there is a substantial interval (>6–12 months) between the completion of that therapy and relapse, the patient's probability of response to subsequent therapies will be very similar to that of a patient who had not had prior therapies. On the other hand, if this interval is short, the patient's probability of response will be very similar to that of a patient who has received prior treatment from metastatic disease.

Most of our observations concerning the treatment of patients with metastatic disease were made in the years prior to the widespread use of adjuvant therapies. At the present time our data base for this new group of patients, which now probably constitute the majority of patients with metastatic disease, is very limited.

6. Utilization of trial results

The standard treatments should be based on results of randomized clinical trials. Subset analyses – especially retrospective subset analyses – should be used with caution and confirmed in prospective controlled clinical trials.

7. General

Today there is a substantial increase in the variety of therapies available to treat patients with metastatic breast cancer. All of these patients will finally succumb to their disease. For this reason we place great emphasis on the importance of continuing exploration for new forms of therapy, new modalities of therapy and new ways of delivering conventional therapy and we urge physicians to enrol their patients in a clinical trial whenever possible and appropriate.

The participants of the Consensus Development Conference

Conference participants

Prof. Dr. med. G. Bastert
Universitäts-Frauenklinik
Homburg/Saar/FRG

Prof. Dr. med. K. W. Brunner
Inselspital
Bern/Switzerland

Ass. Prof. Dr. med. R. C. Coombes
St. George's Hospital
London/GB

Prof. Dr. med. W. Eiermann
Universitäts-Frauenklinik
Klinikum Großhadern
München/FRG

Dr. rer. nat. E. Enghofer
Lederle GmbH & Co
Wolfratshausen/FRG

Prof. Dr. med. I. C. Henderson
Dana-Farber Cancer Institute
Boston/USA

Prof. Dr. med. J. Hilfrich
Gynäkologische Klinik
Krankenhaus Oststadt
Hannover/FRG

Prof. Dr. med. D. K. Hossfeld
Med. Universitätsklinik
Krankenhaus Eppendorf
Hamburg/FRG

Dr. med. F. Jänicke
Klinikum r. d. Isar
München/FRG

Prof. Dr. med. W. Jonat
Universitäts-Frauenklinik
Krankenhaus Eppendorf
Hamburg/FRG

PD Dr. med. M. Kaufmann
Universitäts-Frauenklinik
Heidelberg/FRG

Prof. Dr. med. H. Maass
Universitäts-Frauenklinik
Krankenhaus Eppendorf
Hamburg/FRG

Dr. med. V. Maaßen
I. Universitäts-Frauenklinik
München/FRG

Dr. med. E. Merkle
Universitäts-Frauenklinik
Erlangen/FRG

Prof. Dr. med. A. Neiß
Institut für Biostatistik
und Dokumentation
der Universität
Innsbruck/Austria

Prof. Dr. med. A. Pfleiderer
Universitäts-Frauenklinik
Freiburg/FRG

PD Dr. med. K. Possinger
III. Med. Klinik
Klinikum Großhadern
München/FRG

Ass. Prof. Dr. med. C. Rose
Odense University Hospital
Odense/Denmark

Dr. med. H. Schmid
Universitäts-Frauenklinik
Heidelberg/FRG

Prof. Dr. med. K. D. Schulz
Zentrum für Frauenheilkunde
der Universität
Marburg/FRG

Prof. Dr. med. I. Smith
Royal Marsden Hospital
London/GB

Prof. Dr. med. W. Wilmanns
III. Med. Klinik
Klinikum Großhadern
München/FRG